Diet and Disease

Diet and Disease

Nutrition for Heart Disease, Diabetes, and Metabolic Stress

Katie Ferraro, MPH, RD, CDE

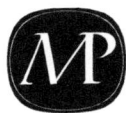

MOMENTUM PRESS
HEALTH

Diet and Disease: Nutrition for Heart Disease, Diabetes, and Metabolic Stress

First published in 2016 by
Momentum Press, LLC
222 East 46th Street, New York, NY 10017
www.momentumpress.net

ISBN-13: 978-1-60650-733-9 (print)
ISBN-13: 978-1-60650-734-6 (e-book)

Momentum Press Nutrition and Dietetics Practice Collection

DOI: 10.5643/9781606507346

Cover and interior design by S4Carlisle Publishing Services Private Ltd., Chennai, India

First edition: 2016

10 9 8 7 6 5 4 3 2 1

Printed in the United States of America.

Abstract

"Let food be thy medicine and medicine be thy food."

—Hippocrates

Can food really take the place of medicine? While modern medicine certainly has its place and does more than its fair share of good, there is no denying that many of society's most perilous chronic diseases are exacerbated by poor diets. Whereas infectious diseases used to cause the most number of deaths, the impact of chronic diseases now far overshadows that of infectious diseases. Diet plays a significant role in the development of a number of types of chronic disease, such as heart disease, diabetes, and certain types of cancer. This title explores the impact of dietary choices on the prevention, management, and treatment of a number of medical conditions and disease states including cardiovascular disease, diabetes and metabolic stress, critical illness, cancer, and HIV/AIDS. Conditions of the gastrointestinal tract, musculoskeletal disorders, rheumatic disease, anemias, hepatobiliary, gallbladder, pancreatic and kidney diseases are covered in the subsequent title *Diet and Disease II*.

Keywords

Medical nutrition therapy, diet and disease, nutrition care process, diet therapy, diabetes, diabetic diet, metabolic stress, heart disease, heart healthy diet

Contents

List of Tables

CHAPTER 1

Nutrition and Heart Disease

Chapter Abstract

Heart disease is the number one killer of Americans, killing about 610,000 people per year, and it is responsible for nearly one in every four deaths in the United States (CDC, 2015). It is also the leading killer of people around the world, accounting for more than 17 million deaths each year. Heart disease does not discriminate, as it is the leading cause of death for both males and females as well as for blacks, Hispanics, and whites (Minino et al. 2011). In addition to its human toll, heart disease also carries a significant financial impact. The American Heart Association has estimated that in 2011, heart disease, hypertension, stroke, and other cardiovascular disease combined accounted for more than $320 billion in direct health care expenditures and annual lost productivity (Mozaffarian et al. 2015).

Despite the bleak mortality statistics and financial impact, the cardiovascular disease (CVD) arena does present many opportunities for nutrition practitioners and health care professionals to affect positive change. Diet and lifestyle play important roles in the prevention and treatment of heart disease, working not only to help reduce the risk of developing heart disease, but also to lower the risk of death from heart disease and the incidence of nonfatal heart attacks as well as the need to undergo serious life threatening interventions (CDC, 2015). This chapter explores the evidence-based guidelines governing current practices about diet and the development, management, and treatment of heart disease.

Preventing Heart Disease

Risk factors for heart disease can be either modifiable or nonmodifiable in nature. Nonmodifiable risk factors are those that you are born with and cannot be changed. These include increasing age, male sex (gender) and heredity (including race). The American Heart Association affirms that the majority of those who die of coronary heart disease are 65 or older. Men are at a greater risk of having heart attacks than are women, and they tend to have heart attacks earlier in life. Children of parents who have heart disease are themselves more likely to develop the disease, and African Americans (because of severe high blood pressure risk) have a higher risk of disease. The risk is also higher among Mexican Americans, American Indians, native Hawaiians and some Asian Americans (AHA, 2015).

While individuals cannot do anything to alter their advancing age or family history (the nonmodifiable risk factors), the modifiable risk factors can be manipulated with diet, exercise, and lifestyle improvements. For those who are at risk of developing heart disease, nutrition therapy can minimize the modifiable risk factors. Modifiable risk factors for heart disease include smoking, elevated blood pressure, elevated blood cholesterol, overweight and obesity, a sedentary lifestyle, and poorly controlled diabetes. Table 1.1 outlines the modifiable risk factors and their associated recommendations to lower the overall risk of developing heart disease.

Table 1.1 Lowering modifiable heart disease risk factors (HHS, 2005), (HHS, 2015), (USDA and HHS, 2011)

Heart Disease Risk Factor	Intervention
Smoking	Smoking cessation
High blood pressure	Increase potassium, lower sodium intake, and increase physical activity to help achieve blood pressure of <120/<80 mmHg
High blood cholesterol	Increase dietary fiber (particularly soluble fiber) and decrease saturated fat, *trans* fat and dietary cholesterol to help achieve total cholesterol <200 mg/dl and LDL <160–100 mg/dL
Overweight and obesity	Decrease excessive caloric intake and increase physical activity to lower body mass index (BMI) and waist circumference
Sedentary lifestyle	Engage in regular physical activity to help lower LDL and raise HDL cholesterol levels; children and adolescents should do one hour or more of physical activity every day, most of which should be moderate- or vigorous-intensity aerobic physical activity
Diabetes	Optimal glycemic control to lower overall CVD risk
Excessive alcohol intake	Avoid overconsumption of alcohol, which elevates blood pressure; limit alcoholic drinks to no more than one per day for women and no more than two per day for men

Disorders of Lipid Metabolism

Lipid metabolism disorders refer to elevated low-density lipoprotein (LDL), total cholesterol, and triglyceride levels as well as low high-density lipoprotein (HDL), and other coronary health conditions such as metabolic syndrome and hypertension. The following section presents an overview of the specifics of lipid metabolism disorders and evidence-based guidelines for dietary intervention to manage risk and optimize outcomes.

Hypercholesterolemia

High levels of cholesterol and other blood lipids promote the formation of plaque in the arteries. Plaque accumulates and can result in impeded blood flow, causing ischemia and tissue damage, which is particularly detrimental when the heart and brain vessels are involved. The causes of high levels of serum cholesterol may be attributable to either genetic and/or environmental factors. The environmental or lifestyle causes may be related to excessive intake of saturated fat and *trans* fatty acids, lack of dietary fiber (both soluble and insoluble dietary fiber), excess body weight, and a sedentary lifestyle (Academy of Nutrition and Dietetics 2015). Cholesterol levels are believed to increase with age, particularly in females; this occurs because as women approach menopause, their declining estrogen levels increase blood levels of cholesterol (Grundy 1999).

Lipid Goals

The overarching goal of nutrition therapy in hypercholesterolemia is to improve serum lipid levels while managing and mitigating other risk factors for cardiovascular disease. The hydrophobic (water-fearing) lipids are transported in the blood packaged with lipoproteins. Very-low-density lipoproteins (VLDLs) are comprised of mostly triglyceride and some cholesterol. Of the lipoproteins, VLDLs contain the highest amount of triglycerides. They are synthesized in the liver and work to export fat from the liver to the body's cells. Low-density lipoproteins (LDLs) are made up of fat and protein and are responsible for carrying cholesterol, triglycerides, and other lipids in the blood to various parts of the body. High circulating levels of LDL cholesterol can lead to the clogging of arteries, which is why they are often referred to as the "bad cholesterol." High-density lipoproteins (HDLs) work to remove cholesterol from the cells, returning them to the liver, and are often called the "good cholesterol" (Rader 2004).

Previous guidelines recommended that LDL and non-HDL cholesterol targets be less than 100 mg/dL, or an optimal goal of less than 70 mg/dL. Updated recommendations from the American College of Cardiology and the American Heart Association developed in conjunction with the National Heart, Lung, and Blood Institute deviated from those previous guidelines, citing a lack of underlying scientific evidence for their existence. The new guidelines do not support target LDL cholesterol or non-HDL cholesterol target treatment goals. Rather, individuals are assessed at different levels depending upon risk (Stone et al. 2014). Individuals looking to gauge their own risk for the development of heart disease can access the Heart-Health Risk Assessments from the American Heart Association online at: http://www.heart.org/HEARTORG/Conditions/More/Tools ForYourHeartHealth/Heart-Health-Risk-Assessments-from-the-American-Heart-Association_UCM_306929_Article.jsp.

As always, consultation with a primary care provider is recommended for determining overall risk and recommended interventions.

Interventions to Lower LDL

The general public tends to misrepresent the effect of dietary cholesterol on blood cholesterol levels. It is common to hear, "I have high blood cholesterol so I shouldn't eat cholesterol in my diet." Practitioners are encouraged to clarify that it is more likely to be the amount of saturated and *trans* fatty acids in the diet that will elevate these LDL or "bad" cholesterol numbers. As such, interventions to help lower LDL through dietary changes should be a primary focus of nutrition education regarding heart disease. To lower LDL with dietary interventions, the focus historically has been on limiting total fat to no more than 25 to 35 percent of calories, reducing saturated fat to less than 7 percent of total calories, limiting or eliminating *trans* fat, and restricting cholesterol to less than 200 mg/day (Carson et al. 2004). This eating pattern has the potential to lower LDL cholesterol levels by up to 16 percent and thus reducing the overall risk of developing heart disease (AND, 2015a).

In recent years there has been much controversy surrounding the efficacy of the "limit total fat" message. Numerous studies highlighting the benefits of the Mediterranean diet and lifestyle—a relatively "high fat" (but "good fat") dietary pattern—have showed a potential to decrease heart disease risk. Consumers may be better served by focusing on replacing saturated fats with more healthful unsaturated fats rather than working on lowering overall fat intake, especially when reductions in calories from lowered fat intake are replaced with refined carbohydrates and sugars. The Academy of Nutrition and Dietetics recommends the following nutrition therapy interventions to counteract elevated total and LDL cholesterol:

- Limit intake of saturated fat, *trans* fat, and cholesterol.
- Consume adequate calories to maintain or achieve appropriate weight.
- Replace saturated fat with monounsaturated or polyunsaturated fat.
- Increase intake of omega-3 fatty acids.
- Increase intake of fiber and in particular, soluble fiber (AND 2015).

Saturated Fat

Saturated fat in the diet increases LDL cholesterol levels in the blood. A 1 percent increase in calories from saturated fat can raise LDL cholesterol levels by approximately 2 percent (Expert Panel on Detection, Evaluation, and Treatment of High Blood Cholesterol in Adults 2001). Saturated fats are typically solid at room temperature and are found in animal products such as lard, butter, cheese, whole milk, fatty meats, ice cream, and cream. While many vegetable oils are high in the heart-healthy unsaturated fats, tropical vegetable oils (coconut, palm, and palm kernel oils) are high in saturated fats and should be minimized or avoided.

For individuals with elevated LDL levels, or for those who have or are at the risk of developing heart disease, the American Heart Association recommends a dietary pattern with no more than 5 to 6 percent of calories from saturated fat. That means if you follow a 2,000 calorie diet, no more than 13 grams of saturated fat per day should be consumed (AHA,

2015a). The daily value (DV) on the Nutrition Facts panel is based on 20 grams of saturated fat per day—a good target for those who need to lower saturated fat. Cutting back on meat, cheese, and full fat dairy is a straightforward approach to reduce saturated fat in the diet. Table 1.2 contains information about the top sources of saturated fat among the U.S. population and their saturated fat content.

Table 1.2 NHANES top sources of saturated fat in the United States diet (NCI, 2013)

Ranking	Food Items	Contribution to Saturated Fat Intake (%)	Cumulative Contribution to Saturated Fat Intake (%)	Saturated Fat per Equivalent Serving (g)
1	Regular cheese	8.5	8.5	6 g in 1 oz. cheddar cheese
2	Pizza	5.9	14.4	9 g in 8 oz. serving
3	Grain-based dessert	5.8	20.2	4 g in 3 oz. coffee cake
4	Dairy desserts	5.6	25.8	4 g in ½-cup ice cream
5	Chicken and chicken mixed dishes	5.5	31.2	7 g in one fried chicken leg
6	Sausage, franks, bacon, and ribs	4.9	36.2	5 g in hot dog
7	Burgers	4.4	40.5	11 g in double-patty hamburger
8	Mexican mixed dishes	4.1	44.6	7 g in fast food beef, bean, cheese burrito
9	Beef and beef mixed dishes	4.1	48.7	12 g in 6 oz. slice meatloaf
10	Reduced fat milk	3.9	52.6	3 g in 8 oz. cup

When providing nutrition counseling for a heart-healthy diet using the food label, practitioners can teach patients and clients how to identify grams of saturated; fat per serving and how to track their intake against their daily 20 gram saturated fat budget. Other tips for lowering saturated fat intake include substituting full-fat dairy for nonfat or low-fat (1 percent) milk and dairy foods, choosing leaner cuts of meat prepared without excessive fat, and selecting olive oil or canola oil in lieu of butter, lard, and higher saturated fat oils when possible. Table 1.3 shows the comparison of higher versus lower saturated fat and calorie food choices. Making these small substitutions can help significantly reduce saturated fat and excess calories.

Table 1.3 Substitution ideas for lowering saturated fat and calories

Instead Of...			Try...		
	Saturated Fat	Calories		Saturated Fat	Calories
Whole milk (1 cup)	5 g	150	Nonfat milk (1 cup)	0 g	80
Swiss cheese (1 oz)	5 g	100	Low fat Swiss cheese (1 oz)	1 g	50
70% lean ground beef (3 oz raw)	9 g	280	95% lean ground beef (3 oz raw)	2 g	115
Premium ice cream (1/2 cup)	11 g	270	Sorbet or sherbet (1/2 cup)	0 g	130
Vegetable oil, palm kernel (1 Tbsp)	11 g	115	Canola oil (1 Tbsp)	1 g	115

Saturated Fat and LDL Particle Size

Advances in laboratory technology now allow practitioners to analyze lipoprotein particle size (LDL subfraction); however, no consensus exists on which method or what the standard for measuring particle size should be (Chung et al. 2009). There is some evidence to indicate that the size and not just the sheer number of LDL particles may play a role in affecting cardiovascular disease risk. Small, dense LDL particles are thought to elevate heart disease risk by invading artery walls more readily, in turn contributing to atherosclerosis and plaque accumulation. Additionally, they may be less easily cleared from the bloodstream than are their larger-sized LDL counterparts. On the other hand, large-sized LDL particles are thought to be more benign than small-sized LDL particles and less likely to increase cardiovascular disease risk. Although limited, emerging data indicates that manipulations of sources of dietary fat (e.g., replacing saturated with polyunsaturated) and carbohydrate (e.g., replacing refined carbohydrates with fiber-containing whole grains) may affect particle size, current dietary education practice for lowering cardiovascular disease risk should continue to focus on lowering overall dietary saturated fat and minimizing refined sugars (Siri-Tarino et al. 2010). While future findings may dictate changes in saturated fat and carbohydrate dietary recommendations for LDL management, there is currently not enough data to warrant such changes in therapy at this time (Ip et al. 2009). A prudent approach to dietary recommendations regarding saturated fat remains to encourage a diet low in overall saturated fat, with an emphasis on reducing animal fats (such as high fat cuts of meat, cheese, and butter) as these are the primary sources of saturated fat in the American diet.

Trans Fat

Trans fatty acids raise LDL cholesterol levels and increase heart disease risk. A 2 percent increase in calories from *trans* fat has been associated with a 23 percent rise in heart disease risk (Ascherio et al. 1994). Findings from the Nurses' Health Study demonstrated that, after adjusting for age and total caloric intake, relative risk of heart disease for those in the quintile that consumed the most *trans* fat was 1.5 times greater than for those in the lowest quintile (Willett et al. 1993). To be fair, the amount of *trans* fat in the general food supply has been reduced dramatically in the past decade; however, consumers are still curious about *trans* fat and practitioners should be prepared to answer questions on minimizing this harmful dietary addition.

There are two general categories of *trans* fats found in the food supply: naturally-occurring and artificial *trans* fats. The primary type of *trans* fat in the U.S. food supply is the artificial kind, prevalent in packaged and processed baked goods, fried foods, and snack items that contain stick margarine or vegetable shortening. *Trans* fats are created by hydrogenating or partially hydrogenating liquid vegetable oils. This process not only transforms liquid to solid fats, but it also enhances the oxidative stability of the fat. Food manufacturers favor *trans* fats due to their extended shelf life and the favorable texture and mouthfeel that *trans* fat-containing foods impart (Remig et al. 2010).

Since 2006, the U.S. Food and Drug Administration (FDA) has required that *trans* fat content of foods be listed on the Nutrition Facts panel. *Trans* fat is listed under the saturated fat on the label and is stated in the nearest 0.5 gram increment when occurring in less than 5 grams per serving, and to the nearest one gram increment when above 5 grams. FDA labeling requirement states that if a food contains less than 0.5 gram *trans* fat per serving (along with total fat less than 0.5 grams per serving and provided that no other claims about fat, fatty acid, or cholesterol content are made), it may be labeled as 0 grams *trans* fat or bear a footnote saying, "Not a significant source of *trans* fat." This "*trans* fat loophole" leads to confusion among consumers who believe they may be eating *trans* fat-free foods, when they actually do contain *trans* fatty acids (as evidenced by the presence of hydrogenated oils in the ingredient list).

Because food manufacturers can determine the serving size labeled on their products, many will purposely use a small serving size in order list the *trans* fat content as zero grams. This gives the consumer a false sense of security, and when the consumer eats multiple portions, they unknowingly consume a significant amount of *trans* fat. Consumers can work to minimize *trans* fat in the diet by looking for the words "partially hydrogenated" when referring to oils in the ingredients list of food labels and avoid these foods when possible. Cutting back on all high fat foods also decreases *trans* fat (and saturated fat) intake. The bottom line is: there is no room for *trans* fat in a heart-healthy diet. The American Heart Association recommends cutting back on foods containing partially hydrogenated vegetable oils in order to reduce *trans* fat in your diet as well as preparing lean meats and poultry without added saturated and *trans* fat (AHA, 2014). The Academy of Nutrition and Dietetics and the *U.S. Dietary Guidelines for Americans, 2010* both maintain that dietary *trans* fat should be limited as much as possible (Academy of Nutrition and Dietetics 2015a), (USDA and HHS, 2011).

Because *trans* fat-containing foods are not consistent with a heart-healthy diet, practitioners should advise patients to reduce or eliminate packaged and processed baked goods, snack items, and fried foods, and to replace them instead with whole grains, fruits, vegetables, nonfat or low-fat dairy, legumes, and lean protein foods. It is also wise to keep in mind that due to growing public interest in limiting *trans* fats, food manufacturers are routinely removing *trans* fats from foods, but replacing the *trans* fats with equally harmful saturated fats. Patients and clients are advised to pay attention to *both* saturated and *trans* fat content of foods and to keep in mind that both work to elevate LDL levels and should be minimized in the diet.

Dietary Cholesterol

While reducing saturated and *trans* fat in the diet is an effective approach to lowering overall and LDL cholesterol, patients with elevated LDL should also keep an eye on, but not become overly concerned about dietary cholesterol intake. Cholesterol originates from two sources: your body and the foods you eat. About three-quarters of blood cholesterol comes from your liver and other cells, while the remaining quarter comes from the foods you eat (AHA, 2014a). Dietary cholesterol is only found in foods that come from animals; thus vegetable-based oils are naturally cholesterol-free. Consumers should not be impressed by French fries fried in "cholesterol-free" vegetable oil as the saturated fat of that oil is the problem, not the cholesterol. Animal-based foods that are high in cholesterol include egg yolks (but not the whites), shrimp, whole milk, and full fat dairy foods, such as butter, cream, and cheese.

Omega-3 Fatty Acids

Omega-3 fatty acids play a role in lowering heart disease risk, not by lowering LDL levels, but rather, by reducing inflammation and preventing the formation of blood clots. Foods that are rich in omega-3 fatty acids include fatty fish (salmon, mackerel, herring, lake trout, sardines, and albacore tuna), and fish oil. Omega-3 fatty acids are also found in some plant foods, such as walnuts, flaxseed, canola, and soybean oils.

The American Heart Association recommends eating fish (particularly fatty fish) at least two times (meaning two servings) per week. According to the American Heart Association, each serving is considered to be 3.5 ounce cooked, or about ¾ cup of flaked fish (AHA, 2015b).

Although the fish supply in the United States is generally considered to be quite safe, the benefits and risks of consuming fish vary depending upon one's life stage. The U.S. Food and Drug Administration advises that children and pregnant women avoid eating fish with the potential for the highest level of mercury contamination. This includes large fish such as shark, swordfish, king mackerel, or tilefish. Pregnant and breast-feeding women and young children are advised to eat 8 to 12 ounces (two to three average servings) per week of fish with potentially lower levels of mercury contamination, such as canned light tuna, salmon, pollock, and catfish (FDA, 2014).

Dietary Fiber

There are two types of dietary fiber: soluble and insoluble fiber. Many fiber containing foods have a similar amount of soluble and insoluble fiber, and individuals should be cautioned to avoid focusing on the *type* of fiber they are eating and to instead concentrate on increasing the *total* amount of dietary fiber. With that said, it may be valuable for some populations to know that it is the soluble fiber that conveys heart health benefits, whereas insoluble fiber is more effective for gastrointestinal health. The goal for individuals at risk for or with established heart disease is 25 to 30 grams of fiber per day. Diets high in fiber and soluble fiber, as components of a cardioprotective diet, have the potential to lower total cholesterol by 2 percent and LDL cholesterol by 7 percent (AND, 2015a).

Soluble fiber, which absorbs water and has a gel-like texture, works to lower CVD risk on two fronts: it increases the excretion of bile acids while at the same time lowering the hepatic synthesis of cholesterol. In plain English, soluble fiber helps remove LDL from your body while it also tells your body internally to make less LDL. For patients with elevated LDL, it may be helpful to liken soluble fiber to a sponge: the fiber soaks up the LDL particles and helps excrete them from the body. It may be helpful to advise patients and clients to think "S" for soluble and "S" for sponge. Good sources of soluble fiber include fruits, vegetables, legumes, and whole grain cereals. Table 1.4 outlines the soluble fiber and total fiber content of some of these foods.

Table 1.4 Total fiber, soluble fiber, and insoluble content of selected foods (USDA-ARS, 2015), (Li, Andrews and Pehrsson 2002), (Quaker Oats Company 2015)

	Serving Size	Total Fiber (g)	Soluble Fiber (g)	Insoluble Fiber (g)
Whole grain cereals				
Bread, whole wheat	1 slice	3	0.7	2.3
Oatmeal, Quaker, quick oats, dry	½ cup	4	2	2
Rice, brown, long grain, cooked	½ cup	1.8	0.2	1.6
Fruit				
Apple, red delicious, raw, ripe with skin	1 medium (3" diameter)	4.4	1.3	3.1
Avocado, raw, California, without skin and seed	½ fruit	4.6	1.7	2.9
Mango, fruit without refuse	1	5.4	2.1	3.3
Vegetables				
Potato, sweet, flesh only	½ cup	4.0 g	1.8	2.2
Broccoli, cooked, boiled, drained, without salt	1 cup	5.1	2.0	3.1
Carrots, cooked, boiled, drained, without salt	1 cup	4.7	1.9	2.8
Legumes				
Red kidney beans, can, drained	½ cup	7.2	1.4	5.8
Lentils, dry, cooked, drained	½ cup	7.8	0.6	7.2

Plant Stanols and Sterols

Plant stanols and sterols are found in small amounts in plant foods. They may be extracted from soybean and tall pine-tree oils and combined in foods with canola oil. In a fashion similar to that of soluble fiber, plant stanols and sterols impede the absorption of cholesterol from the gut, working to lower LDL without raising HDL or triglyceride levels. The American Heart Association suggests that plant stanols and sterols are not for everyone; only individuals who need to lower their cholesterol levels or who have previously suffered from a heart attack may benefit from their inclusion in the diet. Plant stanols and sterols are found in fortified margarine spreads and salad dressings, milk, yogurt, juices, and snack bars. Practitioners are encouraged to advise patients to beware of excess calories from stanol or sterol enhanced foods, keeping in mind that their contribution to unwanted weight gain counteracts the potential cholesterol lowering effects of the plant components.

Interventions to Raise HDL

As seen in the previous section, there are a number of dietary interventions for lowering LDL. Patients and consumers are often disappointed to find that the same does not hold true for elevating HDL. In fact, it is much easier to employ dietary and lifestyle changes to lower high LDL than it is to elevate low HDL. When it comes to HDL, less is more: a higher level of HDL is preferable to a low one. Low HDL elevates one's risk for heart disease and people who have high blood triglycerides also usually have lower HDL. There are a number of factors, including genetics, type 2 diabetes, smoking, being overweight, and being sedentary that can lower HDL cholesterol values (AHA, 2015c). The following interventions may have some limited ability to help elevate low HDL levels.

Niacin

In 2013, a large study addressing the effects of niacin showed that niacin combined with laropiprant does not benefit people at risk for heart disease or stroke and may even prove harmful. The study looked at 25,000 individuals and showed that the drug combination failed to lower the chances of nonfatal heart attack or heart-related death, stroke, or the need for interventions such as angioplasty or bypass surgery. It also could lead to more bleeding, infections, diabetes, and other complications like indigestion and diarrhea, and itchy skin when compared to those taking a placebo (Group 2014). When given in high doses, niacin may also cause an uncomfortable flushing or itching sensation in the face, neck, and upper body area.

Physical Activity

Regular physical activity raises HDL, although the amount of exercise required remains uncertain. Durstine and Thompson have reported that just one intensive exercise session raises HDL (Durstine and Thompson 2001). The *2008 Physical Activity Guidelines for Americans* recommends two and a half hours of moderate-intensity aerobic activity each week (HSS 2008). The evidence-based guidelines of the Academy of Nutrition and Dietetics Evidence Analysis project has found that there is strong/imperative evidence to recommend that "moderate intensity physical activity should be incorporated for at least 30 minutes most, if not all, days of the week, if not contraindicated.... Moderately intense physical activity reduces the risk of CVD events, decreases LDL-C and triglycerides, and increases HDL-C" (Academy of Nutrition and Dietetics 2015a). It should also be noted that U.S. Centers for Disease Control and Prevention (CDC) recommends 150 minutes of physical activity in addition to 2 days of strength training each week (CDC, 2015a). The American Heart Association physical activity guidelines for overall cardiovascular health include:

- At least 30 minutes of moderate-intensity aerobic activity at least 5 days per week for a total of 150, OR
- At least 25 minutes of vigorous aerobic activity at least 3 days per week for a total of 75; or a combination of the two, AND
- Moderate to high intensity muscle-strengthening activity at least 2 days per week for additional health benefits (AHA, 2014)

Alcohol

Moderate alcohol intake is associated with lower heart disease risk as it can raise HDL cholesterol concentrations (De Oliveria E Silva et al. 2000). The exact mechanism by which alcohol raises HDL is unknown. Moderate alcohol intake is defined as no more than one drink per day for women and no more than two drinks per day for men. The American Heart Association defines a serving size of alcohol as a 12-ounce beer, 4-ounce glass of wine, or 1 ounce serving of 80-proof liquor. They encourage patients to be reminded that drinking more alcohol increases dangers such as alcoholism, high blood pressure, obesity, stroke, breast cancer, suicide, and accidents (AHA, 2015d). For individuals who do not currently drink alcohol, taking up drinking just for the HDL effects is not recommended. It is advisable to remind patients that alcohol consumed in excess has a deleterious effect on overall health and increases heart disease risk.

Metabolic Syndrome

The metabolic syndrome (formerly called Syndrome X and also referred to as the insulin resistance syndrome) is a cluster of metabolic abnormalities that increase risk of heart disease and diabetes. Metabolic syndrome currently affects about 34 percent of American adults (AHA, 2015e). The metabolic syndrome was first defined by the World Health Organization in 1998, and it has evolved to include the clustering of three or more risk factors. The four primary risk factors, of which three or more must be present to diagnose, are central obesity, hypertriglyceridemia/low HDL, hyperglycemia, and hypertension. Table 1.5 outlines the inclusion criteria for each risk factor as it pertains to metabolic syndrome.

Excess weight is the primary culprit for metabolic syndrome and as such, reducing and losing excess weight can reduce the associated risks. Overweight and obesity are related to insulin resistance; however, it is the presence of abdominal obesity (the centralized fat that gathers around the mid-region) that increases metabolic risk factors more so than an elevated body mass index. Those with abdominal obesity are sometimes referred to as being apple-shaped, and apple-shaped people tend to be those at higher risk for metabolic syndrome. Pear-shaped individuals amass fat in the buttocks and thighs (as compared to the abdominal) regions.

Table 1.5 Clinical identification of the metabolic syndrome (AHA, 2015e) http://www.uptodate.com/contents/the-metabolic-syndrome-beyond-the-basics

Metabolic Syndrome is Clinically Identified as Any 3 of the Following:
Abdominal obesity as defined by waist circumference
Men: ≥38–41 inches (94–102 cm) Women: ≥32 inches (80 cm)
Triglycerides or HDL Cholesterol
Triglycerides ≥150 mg/dL, or HDL cholesterol in men <40 mg/dL (1 mmol/L) or in women <50 mg/dL (1.3 mmol/L)
Blood pressure
≥130/≥85 mmHg or if you take medicine for high blood pressure
Fasting blood glucose
≥100 mg/dL (5.6 mmol/L)

The treatment for metabolic syndrome involves weight loss, physical activity, dietary improvements, and smoking cessation. According to the Academy of Nutrition and Dietetics guidelines, initial weight loss goals in the treatment of metabolic syndrome should be in the range of 7 to 10 percent of total body weight (Academy of Nutrition and Dietetics 2015a). The American Heart Association emphasizes that treatment of metabolic syndrome involves routinely monitoring body weight, treating individual risk factors, and choosing high blood pressure drugs carefully as they can have varying effects on insulin sensitivity (AHA 2012). With metabolic syndrome, primary goals of treatment are lowering LDL and cholesterol and managing diabetes if present. The secondary goal is to prevent the onset of diabetes in those who have not already developed it (HSS, 2011). If the risk factors persist despite these therapeutic lifestyle changes, practitioners are advised to treat hypertension, to use aspirin for coronary heart disease (CHD) patients and reduce prothrombotic state, and to treat the elevated triglycerides and/or low HDL.

Hypertriglyceridemia

Elevated triglycerides can occur autonomously or alongside elevated blood cholesterol levels. Triglycerides come from food, but the body also produces them. Regardless of the cause or manner of manifestation, hypertriglyceridemia is an independent risk factor for heart disease (Austin, Hokanson and Edwards 1998). Just over one-quarter (25.1 percent) of adults in the United States have elevated triglycerides (>150 mg/dL) (CDC, 2015b). According to National Health and Nutrition Examination Survey (NHANES) data, Mexican-Americans have the highest rates of triglycerides (35.5 percent), followed by non-Hispanic whites (33.2 percent), and African-Americans (15.9 percent) (AHA, 2011). Normal triglyceride levels are below 150 mg/dL and high triglycerides are above 200.

The nutritional management of hypertriglyceridemia is very straightforward: eliminate alcohol, cut back on refined carbohydrate and sugars, increase whole grains and fiber (especially soluble fiber), and exercise or cut calories to achieve and maintain a healthy weight. Omega-3 fatty acids may be helpful in lowering triglycerides in some cases and can be included in the diet from fatty fish and fish oils or as supplements. Supplement with 2 to 4 grams of docosahexaenoic acid (DHA) and eicosapentaenoic acid (EPA), and when possible, utilize prescription drug omega-3 preparations. Prescription omega-3 preparations contain standardized and known amounts of EPA and DHA, whereas over-the-counter omega-3 supplements may not always.

It may occur that when an individual with elevated LDL adopts dietary changes that lower saturated and *trans* fat intake, serum triglycerides will rise. This occurs when the saturated and/or *trans* fat removed from the diet is replaced with sugars or refined carbohydrate. The key to minimizing elevated triglycerides when reducing saturated and *trans* fat intake is to maintain adequate dietary fiber levels. Encourage individuals to aim for 30 grams of fiber per day, with an emphasis on the heart-healthy effects of soluble fiber.

While the goal for triglyceride management remains under 150 mg/dL, the American Heart Association has furthered their recommendations by advocating for a new optimal triglyceride level of 100 mg/dL, although there is currently no data to support the theory that lowering triglycerides to this level is beneficial. Research indicates that replacing saturated fat with unsaturated varieties, engaging in regular physical activity, and losing excess weight can lower triglycerides by 20 to 50 percent (Miller et al. 2011).

If triglycerides are greater than 500 mg/dL, the patient is at increased risk for developing pancreatitis. In this case, the goal is to lower the triglycerides to prevent pancreatitis, adopt a very low-fat diet with less than 15 percent calories from fat, eliminate alcohol, promote weight management and physical activity, initiate fibrate or nicotinic acid, and when triglycerides are lowered under 500 mg/dL, turn to LDL-lowering therapies mentioned above.

Hypertension

Almost 70 million Americans (29 percent)—nearly one in every three adults—have hypertension or high blood pressure. In addition, nearly one in three American adults has prehypertension, which is defined as blood pressure numbers that are higher than normal but not yet in the high blood pressure range. Hypertension costs the U.S. $46 billion per year including the cost to treat and missed days of work (CDC, 2015c). Hypertension is responsible for more than 7 ½ million deaths per year worldwide, accounting for 12.8 percent of total global death, and contributing more than any other individual risk factor (WHO, 2015). Often referred to as "the silent killer", hypertension has no warning signs or symptoms, and most people with high blood pressure are not aware of their condition. The three food and weight-related issues that affect hypertension are excess body weight, high sodium intake, and excessive alcohol consumption (AND, 2015).

Approaches to Lower Blood Pressure

The dietary changes to lower blood pressure include lowering sodium intake, increasing potassium, calcium, and magnesium, and limiting alcohol intake. Lifestyle factors involve increasing physical activity and smoking cessation. The Dietary Approaches to Stop Hypertension (DASH) diet principles are covered at the end of this chapter.

Sodium

There is no question that the majority of people consuming Western consume excessive amounts of salt. The *Dietary Guidelines for Americans, 2010* recommends limiting dietary sodium to no more than 2,300 mg per day. This is restricted even further, to 1,500 mg per day, for African Americans, people 51 years or older, and those who have hypertension, diabetes, or chronic kidney disease (USDA and HHS, 2011). The average daily sodium intake for people ages two and older in the United States is 3,436 mg, and approximately 87 percent of adults eat more than the recommended 2.3 grams of sodium per day (Institute of Medicine 2010), (CDC, 2015d).

Patients and consumers are often unaware of the true sources of sodium in their diet. It is not uncommon to hear, "Oh, I never use salt in my food", or, "We don't even have a salt shaker on the table." Contrary to popular belief, the salt shaker is *not* the primary source of dietary salt in the typical American diet. The majority of salt in the diet comes from packaged, processed, and fast foods. Roughly 77 percent of sodium is from packaged and processed foods purchased at retails stores and restaurants, 5 percent is added to home cooking, 6 percent is added from table salt while eating, and 12 percent comes from naturally occurring sources (Mattes and Donnelly 1991). The impact of sodium from packaged and processed foods is so great and so concentrated that the Centers for Disease Control and Prevention estimate that 44 percent of the sodium we eat comes from only ten different types of foods, listed in Table 1.6 (CDC, 2014). Table 1.7 contains recommendations and information for sodium seasoning alternatives for different types of foods. Table 1.8 provides some tips to reduce salt and sodium intake from the DASH diet. The DASH diet section of this chapter contains more details about lowering salt intake to reduce blood pressure.

Table 1.6 Top 10 sources of sodium in U.S. diet (CDC, 2014)

Top 10 Sources of Sodium Account for 44 Percent of Consumption	
Breads and rolls	Sandwiches
Cold cuts and cured meats	Cheese
Pizza	Pasta dishes
Poultry	Meat dishes
Soups	Snacks

Table 1.7 Seasoning foods without salt (Gerontological Nutritionists 2000)

Type of Food	Salt-free Seasoning Ideas
Asparagus	Garlic, lemon juice, onion, vinegar
Beef	Bay leaf, dry mustard, green pepper, marjoram, fresh mushrooms, nutmeg, onion, pepper, sage, thyme
Bread	Cinnamon, cloves, dill, poppy seed
Broccoli	Lemon juice, garlic
Chicken	Green pepper, lemon juice, marjoram, fresh mushrooms, paprika, parsley, poultry seasoning, sage, thyme, cilantro
Cucumbers	Chives, dill, garlic, onion, vinegar
Fish	Bay leaf, curry powder, dry mustard, green pepper, lemon juice, paprika, bell peppers
Green Beans	Dill, lemon juice, nutmeg, marjoram
Greens	Onion, pepper, vinegar, lemon juice
Lamb	Curry powder, garlic, mint, mint jelly, pineapple, rosemary
Pasta	Basil, caraway seed, garlic, oregano, poppy seed, rosemary
Peas	Green pepper, mint, parsley, onion, fresh mushrooms, garlic
Pork	Apple, applesauce, garlic, onion, sage
Potatoes	Green pepper, mace, onion, paprika, rosemary, parsley, oregano
Rice	Chives, green pepper, saffron, onion
Squash	Cinnamon, nutmeg, mace, ginger
Tomatoes	Basil, marjoram, onion, oregano
Veal	Apricot, cinnamon, cloves, ginger

Table 1.8 Tips to reduce salt and sodium (NHLBI, 2006)

Tips to Reduce Salt and Sodium in Foods	
Condiments	Choose low- or reduced-sodium, or no-salt added versions of foods and condiments when available.
Vegetables	Choose fresh, frozen, or canned (low-sodium or no-salt-added) vegetables.

Tips to Reduce Salt and Sodium in Foods	
Protein	Use fresh poultry, fish, and lean meat, rather than canned, smoked, or processed types.
Cereals	Choose ready-to-eat breakfast cereals that are lower in sodium.
Cured foods	Limit cured foods (like bacon and ham), foods packed in brine (such as pickles, pickled vegetables, olives, and sauerkraut) and condiments (such as mustard, horseradish, ketchup and BBQ sauce). Limit even lower sodium versions of soy sauce and teriyaki sauce as these are often still high in sodium.
Starches	Cook rice, pasta, and hot cereals without salt. Limit instant or flavored rice, pasta, and cereal mixes, which usually have added salt.
Convenience foods	Choose convenience foods that are lower in sodium. Reduce frozen dinners, mixed dishes like pizza, packaged mixes, canned soups or broths, and salad dressing.
Canned foods	Rinse canned foods, such as tuna and canned beans; this removes approximately one-third of the sodium content.
Spices	Use spices instead of salt; flavor foods with herbs, spices, lemon, lime, vinegar, or salt-free seasoning blends.

Potassium

When it comes to providing education about diet and hypertension, firing off lists of what *not* to eat is exhausting! Thankfully, when it comes to lowering blood pressure, you do have a tool in your arsenal that encourages patients to eat *more* of something, and that something is potassium. Emerging research indicates that increasing dietary potassium may be as important as lowering dietary sodium in controlling blood pressure (Houston 2011), (Karppanen, Karppanen and Mervalla 2005), (Suter, Sierro and Vetter 2002). The easiest part about making potassium recommendations is that foods that are high in potassium, such fruits and vegetables, are also naturally low in sodium. In this case, making *one* recommendation works for you on *two* fronts!

The *Dietary Guidelines for Americans, 2010* recommends at least 4.7 grams of potassium per day (USDA and HHS, 2011). In reality, only about 2 percent of U.S. adults meet that guideline (Institute of Medicine 2010). The blood pressure lowering effects of potassium have largely been established based on studies that analyze food-based potassium, as opposed to supplements. As practitioners, we can encourage patients and clients to obtain their potassium from fresh fruits and vegetables, not from supplements. Salt substitutes often contain potassium chloride in place of sodium chloride. Potassium chloride may prove harmful for individuals with kidney problems or who are taking medication for heart, kidney, or liver problems. A safer alternative for sodium substitutes is to stick with commercial salt free seasonings such as Mrs. Dash® or to make your own. Table 1.9 contains a list of herbs and spices, both fresh and dried, to use in lieu of salt when cooking at home. Or make your own salt-free seasoning using the recipe for Spicy Homemade Herb Seasoning listed in Table 1.10 (NIH, 2010).

Table 1.9 Herbs and spices to use in lieu of salt for home cooking (NIH, 2010)

Basil	Crushed red pepper	Paprika/smoked paprika
Ground black pepper	Cumin	Parsley
Cayenne pepper	Garlic	Parsley
Chili powder	Ginger	Rosemary
Cilantro	Mint	Salt-free seasoning mix
Cinnamon	Nutmeg	Tarragon
Coriander	Oregano	Thyme

Table 1.10 Spicy homemade salt-free herb seasoning (AllRecipes.com 2015)

Spicy Homemade Salt-Free Herb Seasoning
Ingredients
1 tsp cayenne pepper
2 Tbsp garlic powder
2 tsp dried basil
2 tsp ground savory
2 tsp onion powder

Spicy Homemade Salt-Free Herb Seasoning
2 tsp dried sage
1 tsp grated lemon zest
2 tsp ground mace
2 tsp dried thyme
2 tsp dried parsley
2 tsp dried marjoram
2 tsp ground black pepper
Instructions
Crush or grind all ingredients together Let stand at least overnight before using Store mixture in an airtight container
Yield
Makes 30, ¾ tsp servings

Alcohol

Alcohol intake has a significant effect on blood pressure (Chen et al. 2008). Moderate alcohol intake, defined as no more than one drink per day for females and no more than two drinks per day for males, decreases the risk of ischemic stroke (USDA and HHS, 2011a). The Academy of Nutrition and Dietetics Evidence Analysis project has found that current evidence does not justify encouraging those who do not drink alcohol to start doing so for any perceived health benefit related to blood pressure and stroke risk. Furthermore, the Evidence Analysis project supports other professional recommendations that alcohol consumption should be limited to no more than two drinks (24 oz. beer, 10 oz. wine, or 3 oz. of 80 proof liquor) per day for most men and no more than one drink per day for women and lighter weight people. This has been shown to result in an approximate systolic blood pressure reduction of 2 to 4 mmHg (Academy of Nutrition and Dietetics 2012), (NHLBI, 2004). Individuals with high blood pressure and greater than moderate alcohol intake are advised to cut back on alcohol or eliminate it entirely from the diet.

Magnesium

In its role as a vasodilator, magnesium intake helps regulate blood pressure. A diet rich in green leafy vegetables, nuts, whole grain breads, and cereals helps assure adequate magnesium intake. For people whose food patterns result in inadequate magnesium intake, dietary supplements to reach 100 percent of the Dietary Reference Intake (DRI) may be indicated. Individuals should be encouraged to meet magnesium needs from increasing variety and quality of their diet, as opposed to obtaining magnesium from supplements (Chobanian et al. 2003).

Calcium

Adequate calcium intake has been positively linked to lowered blood pressure. The Dietary Approaches to Stop Hypertension (DASH) diet (covered in the next section) advocates for the daily inclusion of 2 to 3 servings of nonfat or low-fat dairy products. For those who are unable to tolerate dairy, consider obtaining calcium from other sources such as calcium-fortified soy milk or almond milk, tofu made with calcium salts, canned salmon with bones, or frequent consumption of calcium-rich dark green leafy vegetables. Individuals who consume less than the Recommended Dietary Allowance (RDA) DRI for calcium may consider taking a calcium supplement. The RDA for calcium for males aged 19 to 70 and females aged 19 to 50 is 1,000 mg; the RDA increases to 1,200 mg/day for females aged 51 and older (Institute of Medicine 2010).

Physical Activity

While dietary changes are certainly effective and should be encouraged to lower blood pressure, food is only half the battle. Individuals with hypertension, when not medically contraindicated, should make regular physical activity a part of their efforts to lower blood pressure. Teach patients, and in particular, the "Can't I just take a pill for that?" patients, that exercise can be just as effective at lowering blood pressure as certain medications. Participating in regular aerobic physical activity, such as jogging or brisk walking, for a period of at least 30 minutes per day, 5 days per week lowers blood pressure on average by 4 to 9 mmHg (NHLBI, 2004).

The DASH Diet

The Dietary Approaches to Stop Hypertension (DASH) is a recommended eating pattern based on findings from two large-scale studies conducted by the National Heart, Lung, and Blood Institute. The DASH study findings confirmed that reducing sodium intake along with other dietary and lifestyle changes is an effective therapy for lowering blood pressure. The DASH diet is high in fruits and vegetables and low-fat dairy foods, and low in sodium and saturated fat. It is low in red meat, sweets, and other sugar-sweetened beverages and food. The DASH eating plan includes foods that are good sources of potassium, calcium, magnesium, fiber, and protein. The daily nutrient goals used in the DASH diet (based on a 2,000 calorie diet) are outlined in Table 1.11.

The first DASH study involved 459 adults, 50 percent women and 60 percent African American. The participants were randomly assigned to one of three groups: typical American diet, typical American diet plus more fruits and vegetables, or DASH diet. All of the three groups' sodium levels were about 3,000 mg per day. The results were conclusive: those who ate the typical American diet plus more fruits and vegetables and those who ate the DASH diet plan experienced reduction in blood pressure. The DASH or combination diet groups had reductions in systolic BP of 5.5 mmHg, and diastolic BP was lowered by 3 mmHg.

Table 1.11 DASH diet nutrient goals (NHLBI, 2006)

Nutrient	DASH Diet Daily Goal
Total fat	27% of calories
Saturated fat	6% of calories
Protein	18% of calories
Carbohydrate	55% of calories
Cholesterol	150 mg
Sodium	2,300 mg with 1,500 mg being most effective for lowering BP
Potassium	4,700 mg
Calcium	1,250 mg
Magnesium	500 mg
Fiber	30 g

In the second DASH study, DASH-sodium, 412 participants were randomly assigned to either a typical American diet group or the DASH diet group and then followed for a month as a part of one of three groups of differing sodium levels: 3,000 mg per day, 2,300 mg per day or 1,500 mg per day. The most remarkable reductions in blood pressure were seen at the level of 1,500 mg sodium per day. The 2010 Dietary Guidelines for Americans recommend sodium intake of no more than 1,500 mg sodium per day for African Americans, people aged 51 and older, and those with existing hypertension, diabetes, or chronic kidney disease.

The DASH diet eating pattern was designed to be reflective of commonly available foods. In the event that the study results were positive (which they were), the nutrition recommendations would be easily accessible to the general population. The component of the DASH diet that represents the biggest change for more individuals is the fruits and vegetables component. DASH recommends eating 4 to 5 servings of fruits and 4 to 5 servings of vegetables per day (for a total of 8 to 10 servings of fruits and vegetables per day). This is a remarkably different approach to fruit and vegetable consumption than most patients and most healthy individuals are used to. This level of fruit and vegetable intake provides a significant amount of potassium, with minimal salt and calorie contributions. Further dietary recommendations for the DASH diet include eating 2 to 3 servings of low-fat dairy per day, no more than 2,300 mg sodium per day, weight loss if necessary, and moderate physical activity (at least 3 times per week). This combination of approaches has been shown to lower systolic blood pressure by 4 to 12 mmHg (AND, 2015a). Table 1.12 outlines the food group components of the DASH eating pattern. Table 1.13 offers servings per day in a DASH diet at different calorie levels.

Table 1.12 Sample DASH eating pattern (NHLBI, 2006)

Food Group	Servings per Day	Serving Sizes	Examples & Notes
Grains (with an emphasis on whole grains)	6–8	1 slice bread 1 oz. dry cereal 1/2 cup cooked rice, pasta, or cereal	Whole wheat bread and rolls, whole wheat pasta, English muffin, pita bread, bagel, cereals, grits, oatmeal, brown rice, unsalted pretzels and popcorn

Food Group	Servings per Day	Serving Sizes	Examples & Notes
Vegetables	4–5	1 cup raw leafy vegetable 1/2 cup cut-up raw or cooked vegetable 1/2 cup vegetable juice	Broccoli, carrots, collards, green beans, green peas, kale, lima beans, potatoes, spinach, squash, sweet potatoes, tomatoes
Fruits	4–5	1 medium fruit 1/4 cup dried fruit 1/2 cup fresh, frozen, or canned fruit 1/2 cup fruit juice	Apples, apricots, bananas, dates, grapes, oranges, grapefruit, grapefruit juice, mangoes, melons, peaches, pineapples, raisins, strawberries, tangerines
Fat-free or low-fat dairy	2–3	1 cup milk or yogurt 1 1/2 oz. cheese	Fat-free (skim) or low-fat (1%) milk or buttermilk, fat-free, low-fat, or reduced-fat cheese, fat-free or low-fat regular or frozen yogurt
Lean meat, fish, or poultry	6 or less	1 oz. cooked meats, poultry, or fish 1 egg (limit egg yolk intake to no more than 4 per week)	Select only lean; trim away visible fats; broil, roast, or poach; remove skin from poultry
Nuts, seeds, or legumes	4–5 per week	1/3 cup or 1 1/2 oz. nuts 2 Tbsp peanut butter 2 Tbsp or 1/2 oz seeds 1/2 cup cooked legumes (dry beans and peas)	Almonds, hazelnuts, mixed nuts, peanuts, walnuts, sunflower seeds, peanut butter, kidney beans, lentils, split peas
Fats and oils	2–3	1 tsp soft margarine 1 tsp vegetable oil 1 Tbsp mayonnaise 2 Tbsp salad dressing	Soft margarine, vegetable oil (such as canola, corn, olive, or safflower), low-fat mayonnaise, light salad dressing
Sweets and added sugar	5 or less per week	1 Tbsp sugar 1 Tbsp jelly or jam 1/2 cup sorbet, gelatin 1 cup lemonade	Fruit-flavored gelatin, fruit punch, hard candy, jelly, maple syrup, sorbet and ices, sugar

Table 1.13 DASH eating plan for different calorie levels (NHLBI, 2006)

Calorie Level	Servings per Day		
	1,600 per day	2,000 per day	3,100 per day
Grains	6	10–11	12–13
Vegetables	3–4	5–6	6
Fruits	4	5–6	6
Fat-free or low-fat dairy	4	5–6	6
Lean meat, fish or poultry	2–3	3	3–4
Nuts, seeds or legumes	3/week	1	1
Fats and oils	2	3	4
Sweets and added sugar	0	≤2	≤2

References

Academy of Nutrition and Dietetics. 2015. "Cardiovascular Disease." *Nutrition Care Manual.* http://www.nutritioncaremanual.org. Accessed August 2, 2015.

___. 2015a. "Disorders of Lipid Metabolism, Evidence-Based Nutrition Practice Guidelines, Executive Summary of Guidelines." *Evidence Analysis Library.* http://andevidencelibrary.com. Accessed August 2, 2015.

___. 2012. "Recommendations Summary Hypertension (HTN) Alcohol Consumption." *Evidence Analysis Library.* http://www.andevidence library.com. Accessed August 2, 2015.

AllRecipes.com. 2015. *Spicy Herb Seasoning.* http://allrecipes.com /recipe/spicy-herb-seasoning/detail.aspx. Accessed September 14, 2015

American Heart Association. 2015. *Understand Your Risk of Heart Attack.* http://www.heart.org/HEARTORG/Conditions/HeartAttack/Under standYourRiskofHeartAttack/Understand-Your-Risk-of-Heart-Attack_UCM_002040_Article.jsp. Accessed September 14, 2015.

___. 2015a. *Saturated Fats.* http://www.heart.org/HEARTORG/Gett ingHealthy/NutritionCenter/HealthyEating/Saturated-Fats_UCM_ 301110_Article.jsp. Accessed September 14, 2015.

___. 2015b. *Fish and Omega-3 Fatty Acids.* http://www.heart.org/HEARTORG/GettingHealthy/NutritionCenter/HealthyDietGoals/Fish-and-Omega-3-Fatty-Acids_UCM_303248_Article.jsp. Accessed September 14, 2015.

___. 2015c. *What Your Cholesterol Levels Mean.* http://www.heart.org/HEARTORG/Conditions/Cholesterol/AboutCholesterol/What-Your-Cholesterol-Levels-Mean_UCM_305562_Article.jsp. Accessed September 14, 2015.

___. 2015d. *Alcohol and Heart Health.* http://www.heart.org/HEARTORG/GettingHealthy/NutritionCenter/HealthyEating/Alcohol-and-Heart-Health_UCM_305173_Article.jsp. Accessed September 14, 2015.

___. 2015e. *About Metabolic Syndrome.* http://www.heart.org/HEARTORG/Conditions/More/MetabolicSyndrome/About-Metabolic-Syndrome_UCM_301920_Article.jsp. Accessed September 14, 2015.

___. 2014. *Trans Fat.* http://www.heart.org/HEARTORG/GettingHealthy/NutritionCenter/HealthyEating/Trans-Fats_UCM_301120_Article.jsp. Accessed September 14, 2015.

___. 2014a. *About Cholesterol.* http://www.heart.org/HEARTORG/Conditions/Cholesterol/AboutCholesterol/About-Cholesterol_UCM_001220_Article.jsp. Accessed August 2, 2015.

___. 2014b. *Numbers that Count for a Healthy Heart.* http://www.heart.org/HEARTORG/Conditions/More/ToolsForYourHeartHealth/Numbers-That-Count-for-a-Healthy-Heart_UCM_305427_Article.jsp. Accessed September 14, 2015.

___. 2012. "What is Metabolic Syndrome?" http://www.heart.org/idc/groups/heart-public/@wcm/@hcm/documents/downloadable/ucm_300322.pdf. Accessed September 14, 2015.

___. 2011. "Top Ten Things to Know About Triglycerides and Cardiovascular Disease." http://my.americanheart.org/idc/groups/ahamah-public/@wcm/@sop/@smd/documents/downloadable/ucm_425989.pdf. Accessed September 14, 2015.

Ascherio, A, CH Hennekens, JE Buring, C Master, MJ Stampfer, and WC Willett. 1994. "Trans-fatty acids intake and risk of myocardial infarction." *Circulation* 89: 94–101.

Austin, MA, JE Hokanson, and KL Edwards. 1998. "Hypertriglycer-idemia as a cardiovascular risk factor." *Am J Cariol* 81: 7B–12B.

Carson, JAS, SM Grundy, L Van Horn, N Stone, A Binkoski, and P Kris-Etherton. 2004. "Medical nutrition therapy for the preven-tion and management of coronary heart disease." In *Cardiovascular Nutrition: Disease Prevention and Management*, by JAS Carson, F Burke, and L Hark, 109–148. Chicago, IL: American Dietetic Association.

Centers for Disease Control and Prevention. 2015. "Heart Disease." *Heart Disease Facts.* http://www.cdc.gov/heartdisease/facts.htm. Ac-cessed September 14, 2015.

____. 2015a. *How much physical activity do adults need?* http://www.cdc .gov/physicalactivity/everyone/guidelines/adults.html. Accessed Au-gust 2, 2015.

____. 2015b. *Trends in Elevated Triglycerides in Adults 2001–2012.* http://www.cdc.gov/nchs/data/databriefs/db198.htm. Accessed Sep-tember 14, 2015.

____. 2015c. *High Blood Pressure.* http://www.cdc.gov/bloodpressure /facts.htm. Accessed September 14, 2015.

____. 2015d. *Most Americans Should Consume Less Sodium.* http:// www.cdc.gov/salt/index.htm. Accessed August 2, 2015.

____. 2014. *Top 10 Sources of Sodium.* http://www.cdc.gov/salt/sources .htm. Accessed September 15, 2015.

Chen, L, G Davey Smith, RM Harbord, and SJ Lewis. 2008. "Alcohol intake and blood pressure: a systematic review implementing a Mendelian randomization approach." *PLoS Med* 4(5(3)): e52.

Chobanian, AV, GL Bakris, HR Black, WC Cushman, LA Green, JL Jr Izzo, DW Jones et al. 2003. "The Seventh Report of the Joint Na-tional Committee on Prevention, Detection, Evaluation, and Treatment of High Blood Pressure: the JNC 7 report." *Journal of the American Medical Association* 289(19): 2560–72.

Chung, M, AH Lichtenstein, S Ip, J Lau, and EM Balk. 2009. "Compa-rability of methods for LDL subfraction determination: A systematic review." *Atherosclerosis* 205(2): 342–8.

De Oliveria E Silva, ER, D Foster, Harper, M McGree, CE Seldman, JD Smith, JL Breslow, and EA Brinton. 2000. "Alcohol consumption raises HDL cholesterol levels by increasing the transport rate of apolipoproteins A-I and A-II." *Circulation* 102(19): 2347–52.

Durstine, JL and PD THompson. 2001. "Exercise in the treatment of lipid disorders." *Cardiol Clin* 19: 471–488.

Expert Panel on Detection, Evaluation, and Treatment of High Blood Cholesterol in Adults. 2001. "Executive summary of the Third Report of the National Cholesterol Education Program (NCEP) Expert Panel on Detection, Evaluation, and Treatment of High Blood Cholesterol in Adults (Adult Treatment Panel III)." *JAMA* 285: 2486–2497.

Gerontological Nutritionists. 2000. "Gerontological Nutritionists." *Diet and Disease*. http://www2.fiu.edu/~gn/Resources/DietandDisease.htm. Accessed January 13, 2013.

Group, The HPS2-THRIVE Collaborative. 2014. "Effects of Extended-Release Niacin with Laropiprant in High-Risk Patients." *N Eng J Med* 371: 203–212.

Grundy, SM. 1999. "Nutrition and diet in the management of hyperlipidemia and atherosclerosis." In *Modern Nutrition in Health and Disease*, by ME Shils, JA Olson, M Shike, and AC Ross, 1199–1216. Baltimore, MD: Williams & Wilkins.

Houston, MC. 2011. "The importance of potassium in managing hypertension." *Curr Hypertens Rep* 13(4): 309–17.

Institute of Medicine. 2010. *A Population-Based Policy and Systems Change Approach to Prevent and Control Hypertension*. Board on Population Health and Public Health Practice, National Academy of Sciences.

____. 2010a. *Dietary Reference Intakes for Calcium and Vitamin D*. Washington, DC: National Academies Press.

Ip, S, AH Lichtenstein, M Chung, J Lau, and EM Balk. 2009. "Systematic review: association of low-density lipoprotein subfractions with cardiovascular outcomes." *Annals of Internal Medicine* 7(150(7)): 474–84.

Karppanen, H, P Karppanen, and E Mervalla. 2005. "Why and how to implement sodium, potassium, calcium, and magnesium changes in food items and diets?" *J Hum Hypertens* 19(Suppl 3): S10–9.

Li, BW, KW Andrews, and PR Pehrsson. 2002. "Individual Sugars, Soluble, and Insoluble Dietary Fiber Contents of 70 High Consmption Foods." *Journal of Food Composition and Analysis* 15(6): 715–23.

Mattes, RD and D Donnelly. 1991. "Relative contributions of dietary sodium sources." *J Am Coll Nutr* 10(4): 383–93.

Miller, M, NJ Stone, C Ballantyne, V Bittner, MH Criqui, HN, Goldberg, AC Ginsberg, WJ Howard et al. 2011. "Triglycerides and Cardiovascular Disease: A Scientific Statement From the American Heart Association." *Circulation* 123: 2292–2333.

Minino, AM, SL Murphy, J Xu, and KD Kochanek. 2011. "Deaths: Final data for 2008." *National Vital Statistics Reports* (National Center for Health Statistics) 59(10).

Mozaffarian, D, EJ Benjamin, AS Go, DK Arnett, MJ Blaha, M Cushman, S de Ferranti et al. 2015. "Heart disease and stroke statistics--2015 update: a report from the American Heart Association." *Circulation* 131(1): (4):E:29–322.

National Cancer Institute. 2013. "Risk Factor Monitoring and Methods." *Top Food Sources of Saturated Fat among U.S. Population, 2005–2006 NHANES.* 18-October. riskfactor.cancer.gov/diet/foodsources/sat_fat/sf.html. Accessed August 3, 2015.

National Heart, Lung, and Blood Institute. 2004. JNC 7 Complete Report: The Science Behind the New Guidelines. The Seventh Report of the Joint National Committee on Prevention, Detection, Evaluation, and Treatment of High Blood Pressure - Complete Report.

National Heart, Lung, and Blood Institute. 2006. "Your Guide to Lowering Your Blood Pressure With DASH." *DASH Diet.* www.nhlbi.nih.gov/health/public/heart/hbp/dash/new_dash.pdf. Accessed January 13, 2013.

National Institutes of Health. 2010. "Tasty Stand-Ins for Salt." *NIH Medline Plus*, Spring/Summer: 15.

Quaker Oats Company. 2015. *Quick Oats.* http://www.quakeroats.com/products/hot-cereals/quick-oats.aspx. Accessed August 3, 2015.

Rader, DJ. 2004. "Lipoprotein metabolism." In *Cardiovascular Nutrition: Disease Prevention and Management*, by JAS Carson, FM Burke and LA Hark. Chicago, IL: American Dietetic Association.

Remig, V, B Franklin, S Margolis, G Kostas, T Nece, and JC Street. 2010. "Trans fats in America: a review of their use, consumption, health implications, and regulation." *J Am Diet Assoc* 110(4): 585–592.

Siri-Tarino, PW, Q Sun, FB Hu, and RM Krauss. 2010. "Saturated fat, carbohydrate, and cardiovascular disease." American Journal of *Clinical Nutrition* 91(3): 502–9.

Stone, NJ, J Robinson, AH Lichtenstein, CNB Merz, CB Blum, RH Eckel, AC Goldberg et al. 2014. "2013 ACC/AHA Guideline on the Treatment of Blood Cholesterol to Reduce Atherosclerotic Cardiovascular Risk in Adults." *Circulation* 129(25 (Suppl 2)): S1–45.

Suter, PM, C Sierro, and W Vetter. 2002. "Nutritional factors in the control of blood pressure and hypertension." *Nutr Clin Care* 5(1): 9–19.

U.S. Department of Agriculture - Agricultural Research Service. 2015. *National Nutrient Database for Standard Reference.* http://ndb.nal.usda.gov/ndb/foods/list. Accessed August 3, 2015.

U.S. Department of Agriculture and U.S. Department of Health and Human Services. 2011. *Dietary Guidelines for Americans, 2010, 7th ed.* Washington, DC: U.S. Government Printing Office. http://health.gov/dietaryguidelines/. Accessed April 23, 2012.

___. 2011a. "Report of the Dietary Guidelines Advisory Committee on the Dietary Guidelines for Americans, 2010."

U.S. Department of Health and Human Services. 2015. "Physical Activity Guidelines for Americans." *At-A-Glance: A Fact Sheet for Professionals.* http://www.health.gov/paguidelines/factsheetprof.aspx. Accessed September 18, 2015.

___. 2011. *National Institutes of Health, National Heart Lung and Blood Institute.* http://www.nhlbi.nih.gov/health/health-topics/topics/ms/treatment. Accessed September 15, 2015.

___. 2008. *Physical Activity Guidelines for Americans.* http://health.gov/paguidelines/faqs.aspx. Accessed April 25, 2012.

___. 2005. *Your Guide to Lowering Your Cholesterol with TLC.* National Heart, Lung, and Blood Institute, National Institutes of Health, Bethesda, MD: NIH.

U.S. Food and Drug Administration. 2014. *Fish: What Pregnant Women and Parents Should Know.* June. http://www.fda.gov/Food/FoodborneIllness Contaminants/Metals/ucm393070.htm. Accessed September 14, 2015.

Willett, WC, MJ Stampfer, JE Manson, GA Colditz, FE Speizer, BA Rosner, LA Sampson, and CH Hennekens. 1993. "Intake of trans fatty acids and risk of coronary heart disease among women." *Lancet* 341: 581–585.

World Health Organization. 2015. *Raised blood pressure.* http://www.who.int/gho/ncd/risk_factors/blood_pressure_prevalence_text/en/. Accessed September 15, 2015.

CHAPTER 2

Nutrition and Diabetes

Chapter Abstract

Diabetes is a metabolic disease characterized by disruptions in blood glucose regulation. Diabetes may be a result of the pancreas not producing insulin (as seen in type 1 diabetes), or the body's inability to properly use the insulin that is produced (which occurs in type 2 diabetes). In the United States, more than 29 million people, or about 9.3 percent of the population, have diabetes; and one out of four of these people do not know that they have the disease. Of the diagnosed cases of diabetes, 5 percent have type 1 diabetes and 95 percent have type 2 diabetes (ADA, 2014). The majority of the people with type 2 diabetes are overweight or obese. Being overweight or obese makes it more difficult for the body to utilize insulin produced by the pancreas to shuttle sugar into the body's cells. In people with type 2 diabetes, losing weight helps shrink fat cells, which in turn can improve the body's ability to produce and effectively use insulin.

Diabetes has a massive effect at both the individual health level and the greater health care system level. Having diabetes puts an individual at a 50 percent higher risk of death in adulthood. People with diabetes are at increased risk of developing a number of health-related side effects, including:

- Blindness
- Kidney failure
- Heart disease
- Stroke
- Loss of toes, feet, or legs (amputation)

From a financial standpoint, medical costs are more than twice as high for someone with diabetes as compared to someone without diabetes. The financial impact of diabetes results in $245 billion in total medical costs and lost work and wages for those diagnosed with the disease (ADA, 2014).

The Role of Medical Nutrition Therapy for Diabetes

Medical Nutrition Therapy (MNT) is considered to be the most important component for the treatment of diabetes mellitus (Kodama et al. 2009). MNT plays a critical role in preventing diabetes, managing existing diabetes, and preventing or reducing the potential complications related to poor glycemic, lipid, and blood pressure control. According to the American Diabetes Association (ADA) Nutrition Recommendations and Interventions for Diabetes Position Statement, MNT is important at all levels of diabetes prevention:

- *Primary prevention*: to prevent diabetes with the use of MNT and public health intervention in those with obesity and pre-diabetes;
- *Secondary prevention*: to prevent complications with the use of MNT for metabolic control of diabetes, type 1, type 2, and gestational;
- *Tertiary prevention*: to prevent morbidity and mortality with the use of MNT to delay and manage complications of diabetes, type 1, and type 2.

MNT provided by a registered dietitian nutritionist (RD/RDN) is recommended by both the ADA and the Academy of Nutrition and Dietetics (AND) for individuals with prediabetes, type 1, and type 2 diabetes, as well as for populations affected by metabolic and glycemic disruption (AND, 2011), (ADA, 2015). It is recommended that an RDN knowledgeable and skilled in MNT be the team member who plays the leading role in providing nutrition care; however, it is important that all team members and practitioners be knowledgeable about MNT for diabetes and support its implementation (Franz et al. 2010).

Goals of Medical Nutrition Therapy for Diabetes Mellitus

For individuals at risk for diabetes or with prediabetes, MNT goals are to decrease the risk of diabetes and cardiovascular disease (CVD) by promoting healthy food choices and physical activity leading to moderate weight loss that can be successfully maintained. Although the etiologies of type 1 and type 2 diabetes differ, MNT goals for both are similar:

1. To promote and support healthful eating patterns, emphasizing a variety of nutrient-dense foods in appropriate portion sizes in order to improve overall health and specifically to:
   - Attain individualized glycemic, blood pressure, and lipid goals
   - Achieve and maintain body weight goals
   - Delay or prevent complications of diabetes
2. To address individual nutrition needs based on personal and cultural preferences, health literacy and numeracy, access to healthful food choices, willingness and ability to make behavioral changes, and barriers to change
3. To maintain the pleasure of eating by providing positive messages about food choices while limiting food choice only when indicated by scientific evidence
4. To provide the individual with diabetes practical tools for day-to-day meal planning rather than focusing on individual macronutrients, micronutrients, or single foods (ADA, 2015)

Diabetes Risk Factors

Type 1 diabetes is a genetic condition that is usually diagnosed in children and young adults. Because people with type 1 diabetes do not produce insulin, they must inject insulin daily to help transport the sugar from foods into the body's cells. The risk factors for type 1 diabetes are not fully understood; however, having a family member who has type 1 slightly increases the risk of developing the disease. Some environmental factors and exposure to viral infections have been linked to increased risk for the development of type 1 diabetes (IDF, 2014).

Type 2 diabetes is characterized by **insulin resistance**, which is the body's inability to use insulin properly. Risk factors for type 2 diabetes include:

- Being overweight and/or physically inactive
- Having a family history of diabetes
- Having diabetes while pregnant or a history of poor nutrition during pregnancy
- African Americans, Mexican Americans, American Indians, Native Hawaiians, Pacific Islanders, and Asian Americans are at higher risk for diabetes
- Smoking
- Increasing age
- High blood pressure (IDF, 2014)

There are a number of online tools available to patients to help assess their diabetes risk. The American Diabetes Association has a type 2 diabetes risk test available at http://www.diabetes.org/are-you-at-risk/diabetes-risk-test/ and the Centers for Disease Control National Diabetes Prevention Program prediabetes risk test can be found at http://www.cdc.gov/widgets/Prediabetes/html5/iframe.html. Prediabetes will be discussed later in the chapter and all people are advised to consult with their primary care provider to discuss risk factors for the development of prediabetes and diabetes.

Diagnosing Diabetes

The American Diabetes Association has established the criteria for the diagnosis of diabetes. The criteria call for the diagnosis of diabetes using the following blood tests and outcome results:

- Hemoglobin A1c (HbA1c) ≥6.5 percent, or
- Fasting plasma glucose (fasting blood glucose) ≥126 mg/dL (7.0 mmol/L) (fasting is defined as no caloric intake for at least 8 hours), or

- Two-hour post prandial glucose (PG) ≥200 mg/dL (11.1 mmol/L) using a glucose load of 75 g anhydrous glucose dissolved in water, or
- In a patient with classic symptoms of hyperglycemia (high blood sugar) or hyperglycemic crisis, a random plasma glucose ≥200 mg/dL (11.1 mmol/L)

The standards state that in the absence of unequivocal hyperglycemia, results should be confirmed by repeat testing (on a separate day) (ADA, 2015a).

HbA1c

The HbA1c is the laboratory test used to assess average blood glucose levels over the preceding two to three months and has been shown to be a strong predictive value for diabetes complications (ADA, 2013). One way to think of HbA1c is that it measures the "stickiness" of the red blood cells—if an individual has chronically high blood sugar, the sugar will result in "stickier" red blood cells and a higher HbA1c value; lower HbA1c values correlate with lower average blood sugar readings. There are a number of mobile applications, websites, and references that can help patients convert their HbA1c to their estimated average glucose levels. One such calculator is available from the American Diabetes Association at http://www.diabetes.org/living-with-diabetes/treatment-and-care/blood-glucose-control/a1c/.

All people with diabetes should receive routine HbA1c testing at initial assessment and as part of continuing care. The frequency of testing HbA1c should be determined by the clinical situation, the treatment method used, and by clinical judgment. The American Diabetes Association recommends the following for HbA1c testing:

- Perform the A1c test at least two times per year in patients who are meeting treatment goals (and who have stable glycemic control).
- Perform the A1c test quarterly in patients whose therapy has changed or who are not meeting glycemic goals.

- Use of point-of-care testing for A1c provides the opportunity for more timely treatment changes (ADA, 2015).

For adults, the American Diabetes Association recommends an HbA1c goal of <7 percent in nonpregnant adults as a way to reduce the long-term risk of microvascular and macrovascular disease. Other providers may counsel on tighter HbA1c control (<6.5 percent) for people who can achieve this level without significant hypoglycemia or other adverse effects of treatment. Less stringent HbA1c goals (such as <8 percent) may be appropriate for those with a history of severe hypoglycemia, limited life expectancy, advanced complications, extensive co-morbid conditions, or long-standing diabetes in whom the general goal is difficult to attain (ADA, 2015).

Hypoglycemia

Hypoglycemia is defined as abnormally low blood glucose levels, usually less than 70 mg/dL. The risk for hypoglycemia increases in older adulthood as a result of renal changes, slowed counter-regulation, inadequate hydration, use of multiple medications, erratic food intake, and slowed intestinal absorption.

Symptoms of Hypoglycemia

Symptoms of hypoglycemia include:

- Shakiness
- Nervousness or anxiety
- Sweating, chills, and clamminess
- Irritability or impatience
- Confusion, including delirium
- Rapid/fast heartbeat
- Lightheadedness or dizziness
- Hunger and nausea
- Sleepiness
- Blurred/impaired vision

- Tingling or numbness in the lips or tongue
- Headaches
- Weakness or fatigue
- Anger, stubbornness, or sadness
- Lack of coordination
- Nightmares or crying out during sleep
- Unconsciousness (American Diabetes Association 2015)

Management of Hypoglycemia

The American Diabetes Association recommends the following for the management of hypoglycemia:

- Individuals at risk for hypoglycemia should be asked about symptomatic and asymptomatic hypoglycemia at each encounter.
- Glucose (15 to 20 g) is the preferred treatment for a conscious individual with hypoglycemia, although any form of carbohydrate that contains glucose may be used.
- Fifteen minutes after treatment, if self-monitoring of blood glucose shows continued hypoglycemia, the treatment should be repeated. One self-monitoring returns to normal, the person should consume a meal or snack to prevent recurrence of hypoglycemia.
- Glucagon should be prescribed for all individuals at increased risk of severe hypoglycemia and caregivers or family members should be instructed on its administration (ADA, 2015).

Depression and cognitive dysfunction may interfere with self-monitoring and total diabetes care management. Visual acuity and fine motor skills can also interfere with self-monitoring of blood glucose; therefore, assistance in choosing the appropriate glucometer to meet the individual's needs may be required. In some cases, use of a talking glucometer may be warranted.

During acute illnesses, increases in counter regulatory hormones occur, and the need for insulin and oral glucose-lowering medications may often be higher than usual. This can lead to the development of hyperglycemia and ketoacidosis. In situations like this, patients should be advised the following (ADA, 2008), (ADA, 2002):

- Test plasma glucose and ketones more often (at least every 2 to 4 hours) and report moderate to large urine ketones to the health care team.
- Increase fluid intake and assure adequate hydration.
- If plasma glucose is <100, take additional carbohydrate containing liquids or food as tolerated (amount of daily carbohydrate sufficient to prevent starvation ketosis is 150 to 200 grams or 45 to 50 grams every 3 to 4 hours). (NOTE: This additional carbohydrate can come from crackers, soup, regular soda or juice, or glucose tablets.)
- Continue insulin and oral glucose-lowering medications.
- Watch for signs of ketoacidosis: nausea, vomiting, abdominal pain, increased drowsiness, fruity odor to breath, cracked lips, cracked mouth, cracked tongue.

Prediabetes

In the United States, one in three, or around 86 million, people have prediabetes. Of these, nine out of 10 do not know they have prediabetes. Having prediabetes makes it much more likely that one will develop diabetes; in fact, 15 to 30 percent of people with prediabetes will develop type 2 diabetes within five years (CDC, 2014). One of the most effective ways to prevent the progression from prediabetes to diabetes is to lose excess weight. As little as 5 to 10 percent body weight loss in an overweight or obese person with prediabetes can help lower the risk for developing diabetes. The American Diabetes Association specifically recommends a target loss of 7 percent of body weight for people with prediabetes in order to prevent or delay type 2 diabetes (ADA, 2015).

Prediabetes Risk Factors

There are a number of factors that increase a person's chance of developing prediabetes. The likelihood of developing prediabetes is elevated if one:

- is aged 45 or older;
- is African American, Hispanic/Latino, American Indian, Asian American, or Pacific Islander;
- has a parent, brother, or sister with diabetes;
- is overweight;
- is physically inactive;
- has high blood pressure or takes medicine for high blood pressure;
- has low HDL cholesterol and/or high triglycerides;
- is a woman who had diabetes during pregnancy;
- has been diagnosed with Polycystic Ovarian Syndrome (PCOS) (ADA, 2014a).

Identifying Prediabetes

According to the American Diabetes Association Standards of Medical Care in Diabetes 2015, asymptomatic adults should be tested for risk for future diabetes (i.e., prediabetes) regardless of age if they are overweight or obese (body mass index ≥25 kg/m² or ≥23 kg/m² in Asian Americans) and have one or more risk factors associated with diabetes. For all patients and in particular those who are overweight or obese, testing should commence at 45 years of age. If the test results are normal, then repeat testing should be carried out at three-year intervals (ADA, 2015). The American Diabetes Association (ADA) calls prediabetes (or impaired glucose tolerance, IGT) a "category of increased risk for diabetes" and says prediabetes or IGT is present when:

- fasting plasma glucose (FPG, i.e., blood glucose) is 100 mg/dL to 125 mg/dL (5.6 mmol/L to 6.9 mmol/L), or
- two-hour post prandial glucose (PG) using an oral glucose tolerance test of 75 g anhydrous glucose dissolved in water is

140 mg/dL to 199 mg/dL (7.8 mmol/L to 11.0 mmol/L), or
- hemoglobin A1c (A1c) is 5.7 to 6.4 percent.

For all three tests, the ADA asserts that risk is continuous, extending below the lower limit of the range of the test and becoming disproportionately greater at higher ends of the range (ADA, 2015).

Prediabetes Management

The American Diabetes Association Standards of Medical Care in Diabetes 2015 sets forth the following recommendations for people with prediabetes in order to prevent or delay the development of type 2 diabetes:

- People with prediabetes should be referred to an intensive diet and physical activity behavioral counseling program targeting loss of 7 percent of body weight and increasing moderate-intensity physical activity (such as brisk walking) to at least 150 minutes/week.
- Follow-up counseling may be important for success and based on the cost-effectiveness of diabetes prevention, such programs should be covered by third-party payers.
- Metformin therapy for prevention of type 2 diabetes may be considered in those with impaired glucose tolerance, impaired fasting glucose, or an HbA1c value of 5.7 to 6.4 percent, especially for those with a body mass index ≥ 35 kg/m^2, aged <60 years, and women with prior gestational diabetes.
- At least annual monitoring for the development of diabetes in those with prediabetes is suggested.
- Screening for and treatment of modifiable risk factors for cardiovascular disease is suggested.
- Diabetes self-management education (DSME) and support (DSMS) programs are appropriate venues for people with prediabetes to receive education and support to develop and maintain behaviors that can prevent or delay the onset of diabetes (ADA, 2015).

Meal Planning for Diabetes

Over the last one hundred years, dietary prescriptions for diabetes have varied widely from the very-low carbohydrate diets initiated before insulin was discovered, to the high-carbohydrate, high-fiber vegan diets often endorsed today by some health professionals. One thing has remained consistent, and that is that dietary prescription for diabetes is and should continue to be centered around carbohydrates. The so-called diabetic diets that were used before exogenous insulin became widely available consisted mainly of protein and fats. The optimal diet for people with diabetes (PWD) (with or without the need for insulin) described by Elliott P. Joslin in 1927 consisted of 100 grams carbohydrate. In the 1920s and early 1930s, normal or even high carbohydrate diets were used by many physicians for treating PWD. From the 1940s, the debate continues with the pendulum swinging back and forth on what is considered to be the best balance of carbohydrate, protein, and fat (Wheeler and Pi-Sunyer 2008). Although it is well known that the restriction of calories is essential for the achievement of adequate glycemic and lipid control, the optimal dietary macronutrient composition for PWD remains controversial (Kodama et al. 2009).

There is no one recommended "diabetes diet" and no one-size-fits-all approach to meal planning for diabetes. In fact, the basic principles of healthy meal planning for diabetes are very similar to how a person *without* diabetes should eat. For someone who is overweight or obese and has type 2 diabetes, cutting back on calories to lose weight can help reduce blood sugar. The American Diabetes Association emphasizes that all people with diabetes should choose a variety of nutrient-dense foods in appropriate portion sizes to improve overall health (ADA, 2015).

Macronutrient Considerations

The proper distribution of calories from carbohydrates, fats, and proteins helps to assure optimal glycemic control while providing adequate, but not excessive, amounts of nutrients. While carbohydrates, proteins, and fats all contribute calories, a person with diabetes should remain most focused on carbohydrate intake, while at the same time not dismissing the importance of protein and fat in meal planning and effect on health.

Contribution of Dietary Carbohydrate

Low-carbohydrate diets have been defined as providing anywhere between 50 to 150 grams carbohydrate per day (Westman et al. 2007). The Dietary Reference Intake (DRI) recommendations state that the minimum amount of carbohydrate that should be consumed by adults is 130 grams per day. Although brain fuel needs can be met on lower-carbohydrate diets, long-term metabolic effects of very-low-carbohydrate diets are unclear (ADA, 2008), (ADA, 2013). A high-protein diet is not recommended for PWD due to the risk of nephropathy (Kodama et al. 2009).

Although low-carbohydrate diets may seem to be the logical approach to lowering postprandial glucose, carbohydrate-containing foods are important sources of energy, fiber, vitamins, and minerals. Carbohydrates also contribute to the palatability of the diet, thereby making them important components of the diet for PWD (ADA, 2013), (ADA, 2008), (Franz et al. 2010).

Carbohydrate Selections.   Carbohydrates are key when it comes to managing glucose (blood sugar) levels. The best sources of carbohydrate are:

- Whole grains and legumes
- Fruits and vegetables
- Low-fat and non-fat dairy foods

The ADA stresses that these types of foods are preferable to other carbohydrate sources, especially those that contain added fats, sugars, or sodium. People with diabetes should avoid sugar-sweetened beverages (like soda). The Acceptable Macronutrient Distribution Range (AMDR) of 45 to 65 percent of calories coming from carbohydrate applies to people with diabetes as well. For someone on a 2,000 calorie diet this equates to 225 to 325 grams of carbohydrate per day. This amount of carbohydrate should be spread out over the day and a minimum of 130 grams (the DRI for carbohydrate) should be achieved. A Registered Dietitian Nutritionist (RD/RDN) or Certified Diabetes Educator (CDE) can help people with diabetes figure out how many grams of carbohydrate per day are right for them, as well as the best way to spread those carbohydrates out over the day.

Table 2.1 Sample distribution of 350 grams carbohydrate

Meal or Snack
Breakfast: ½ cup dry oatmeal (27 g), 1 cup nonfat milk (12 g), ½ cup blueberries (11 g)
Snack: whole wheat pita bread (4 in., 15 g), ½ cup hummus (25 g), cucumber, sliced (4 g), tomato (5 g)
Lunch: 3 oz. curried chicken kabobs (5 g), 1 cup long grain white rice (45 g), 1 cup boiled greens (4 g), 1 glass Indian lassi made with yogurt, sugar, water (21 g)
Snack: 1 mango (31g), ¼ cup almonds (4g), 1 oz. potato chips (15g)
Dinner: ½ cup pinto beans (22 g), 2 corn tortillas (21 g), ¼ cup salsa (4 g), ¼ avocado (3 g), 1 cup squash (10 g), 1 orange (15 g)
Snack: 1 cup ice cream (37 g), ½ banana (13 g), 1 maraschino cherry (1 g)
Total

Carbohydrate Intake Consistency.   Meal and snack carbohydrate intake for a person with type 1, type 2, and gestational diabetes should be consistently distributed throughout the day on a day-to-day basis. Consistency in carbohydrate intake has been shown to result in improved glycemic control in persons receiving either MNT alone, glucose-lowering medications, or fixed insulin doses (Franz et al. 2010). Table 2.1 shows the distribution of 350 grams of carbohydrate over three meals and three snacks.

Dietary Fiber and Diabetes.   Dietary fiber is found in plant foods and can help control blood sugar levels in people with diabetes (Post et al. 2012). Most Americans only eat 10 to 12 grams per day, but the recommendation is to eat 20 to 35 grams of fiber each day (NIH, 2014a). Eating more fruits and vegetables, and choosing whole grains are two great ways to get fiber. To bump up individual fiber intake, one should think in terms of "halves":

- Make half of the plate fruits and vegetables.
- Make half of the grains whole grains.

For more information on meal planning for diabetes, check out the My-FoodAdvisor tool from the ADA available at http://tracker.diabetes.org/.

Contribution of Dietary Fat

The amount of fat people with diabetes should eat is the same as the general, healthy population. Where the fat comes from matters though, and the type of fat is more important than total fat (Estruck, Salas-Salvado and Investigators 2013). One of the easiest ways to select heart-healthy fats is to eat a Mediterranean-style diet. The ADA recommends a Mediterranean-style diet because it is rich in monounsaturated fats, sometimes called "good fat". Sources of monounsaturated fats include:

- Olive oil and canola oil
- Avocados
- Nuts and seeds

All people, whether they have diabetes or not, should look to minimize the amount of saturated fats in the diet. Saturated fats come from foods like butter, meat, and full fat dairy foods.

The Mediterranean Diet. The Mediterranean-style diet incorporates a high monounsaturated fatty acid (MUFA) dietary pattern. A modified Mediterranean diet, in which polyunsaturated fatty acids were substituted for monounsaturated fatty acids, reduced overall mortality in elderly Europeans by 7 percent (ADA, 2008). In a two-year dietary intervention study, Mediterranean and low-carbohydrate diets were found to be effective and safe alternatives to a low-fat diet for weight reduction in moderately obese participants (ADA, 2013). A recent randomized trial looking at high-risk individuals in Spain showed the Mediterranean dietary pattern reduced the incidence of diabetes in the absence of weight loss by 52 percent compared to the low-fat control group (ADA, 2013).

With regards to pancreatic beta-cell health and insulin resistance, fatty acids in monounsaturated oils were found to mitigate the negative effects of saturated palmitic acid on beta-cell death (Franz et al. 2003), and unlike circulating saturated fatty acids, monounsaturated fatty acids do not cause insulin resistance (Chavez and Summers 2003). It would appear from this research that a Mediterranean diet is beneficial for diabetes management; however, a clearer understanding of the protective mechanisms from differing components of the diet is still warranted (Franz et al. 2010).

Trans Fatty Acids. In nondiabetic individuals, reducing trans-fatty acid intake decreases plasma total and LDL cholesterol. Saturated and trans-fatty acids are the principal dietary determinants of plasma LDL cholesterol. Thus, minimal intake of trans-fatty acids is recommended for PWD (ADA, 2008). This can be achieved primarily through minimizing packaged and processed dessert and snack foods that are the primary sources of trans fat in the Western diet.

Saturated Fats. In nondiabetic individuals, reducing saturated fatty acids decreases plasma total and LDL cholesterol. Although reducing saturated fatty acids may also reduce HDL cholesterol, the ratio of LDL cholesterol to HDL cholesterol is not adversely affected (ADA, 2008). The recommendation for saturated fatty acids for PWD is <7 percent of total calorie intake per day. As covered previously, circulating saturated fatty acids appear to cause pronounced insulin resistance (Chavez and Summers 2003). Minimizing saturated fatty acid intake is best achieved through a reduction in animal foods like meats and full fat dairy, tropical oils and other added fats.

Contribution of Dietary Protein

The focus of protein intake for the management of diabetes was originally to preserve lean body mass; although now, dietary protein is believed to play a role in the management of hyperglycemia and body weight (ADA, 2015). Although glucose produced from ingested protein has been shown in a number of studies to produce increases in serum insulin responses, it has not been shown to have an effect on plasma glucose concentration in people with type 2 diabetes (ADA, 2008). Insulin deficiency and insulin resistance may be the cause of abnormal protein metabolism, but they are usually corrected with good glycemic control

(ADA, 2008). Diets with protein content >30 percent of total energy have been shown in small, short-term studies to reduce glucose and insulin concentrations, reduce appetite, and increase satiety. The DRI recommends a macronutrient distribution of protein in the range of 10 to 35 percent of energy intake, with 15 percent being the average adult intake in the U.S. and Canada (ADA, 2008). The RDA is 0.8 grams of good quality protein per kilogram body weight (on average, equating to approximately 10 percent of total calories) (ADA, 2008).

The Glycemic Index

The glycemic index (GI) is a rating system that ranks foods according to their likelihood of raising blood glucose. The glycemic index scale ranges from 0 to 100, with 100 being pure glucose. Lower GI foods cause a lower or more gradual rise in blood sugar compared to high GI foods, which spike blood sugar faster.

While selecting low versus high GI foods may be helpful in regulating blood sugar control in people with diabetes, it is not a preferred therapy, and there are a number of limitations to the GI meal planning approach. There is no widespread agreement about the GI of various foods, and the comparison weight of 50 grams of carbohydrate used to determine a food's GI is not always representative of typical serving sizes. Considering just the GI of a food when considering whether or not to include it in the diet for diabetes may be an oversimplification and may result in the removal of healthful, nutrient-dense foods from the diet. Current recommendations for healthy meal planning with diabetes already encourage food choices that tend to be lower GI options, such as whole grains, legumes, fruits, vegetables, and milk and milk products. Most people with diabetes will find that using the GI to select foods is not the most effective way to regulate blood sugar, and there is no evidence to suggest it is at all helpful in people without diabetes.

Gestational Diabetes

Women who have diabetes in their first trimester are considered to have type 2 diabetes. Gestational diabetes mellitus (GDM) is diagnosed in pregnant women in their second or third trimester when they do not clearly have overt diabetes. Previously, gestational diabetes referred to any degree of glucose intolerance first recognized during pregnancy. This definition has been replaced by the updated trimester-based diagnosis to capture a more precise detection and classification of gestational diabetes (ADA, 2015).

Risk Factors for Gestational Diabetes

Women who are at elevated risk for developing gestational diabetes include those who:

- are aged 25 or older when pregnant;
- are from a high risk ethnic group such as Hispanic American, African American, Native American, Southeast Asian, or Pacific Islander;
- have a family history of diabetes;
- previously gave birth to a baby that weighed more than 9 pounds or had a birth defect;
- have high blood pressure;
- have too much amniotic fluid;
- have had an unexplained miscarriage or stillbirth;
- were overweight or obese prior to pregnancy;
- gain excessive weight during pregnancy;
- have polycystic ovarian syndrome (NIH, 2014b).

Testing for and Diagnosing Gestational Diabetes

Pregnant women with risk factors for diabetes should be tested for undiagnosed type 2 diabetes on their first prenatal visit. Standard diagnostic criteria for diagnosing diabetes are used in this case. Women who were not previously known to have diabetes should be tested for gestational diabetes at 24 to 28 weeks of gestation. Gestational diabetes is diagnosed using either a one-step or two-step strategy. The one-step strategy involves using a 75-gram oral glucose tolerance test (OGTT), with plasma glucose measurements taken at fasting, and at 1 and 2 hours after ingesting the

75-gram glucose load. The OGTT test should be administered in the morning following an overnight fast of at least eight hours. The diagnosis of gestational diabetes is made when any of the following plasma glucose levels are met or exceeded:

- Fasting—92 mg/dL (5.1 mmol/L)
- 1 hour following ingestion of 75 g glucose load—180 mg/dL (10.0 mmol/L)
- 2 hours following ingestion of 75 g glucose load—153 mg/dL (8.5 mmol/L)

The two-step strategy involves performing a 50-gram (nonfasting) screen followed by a 100-gram OGTT for those who screen positive (ADA, 2015).

Physical Activity and Diabetes

Physical activity is a vital component of diabetes prevention and management, as well as for the prevention of potential diabetes complications. At least 2.5 hours of moderate to vigorous physical activity each week should be undertaken to prevent type 2 diabetes onset in high-risk adults (S. Colberg, R. Sigal and B. Fernhall et al. 2010). In addition, epidemiological studies suggest that higher levels of physical activity may also reduce the risk of developing GDM during pregnancy (S. Colberg, R. Sigal and B. Fernhall et al. 2010). Some benefits of physical activity to PWD include (S. Colberg, R. Sigal and B. R. Fernhall et al. 2010):

- Reduction of cardiovascular risk factors
- Promotion of a healthy weight
- Reduction in body weight and body fat
- Improvement in blood glucose control and tolerance
- Increase in peripheral insulin sensitivity
- Reduction in insulin requirements
- Improvement in sense of well-being
- Decrease in stress

Although physical activity is a crucial component of care, the nutrition practitioner must be aware of the individual's potential restrictions for exercise and the metabolic effects and benefits for PWD in order to maximize rewards and minimize risks of injury and poor medical outcomes. In general, PWD who exercise occasionally may require assistance to maintain normal blood sugar levels, by either the adjustment of medications, the amount of food consumed, the timing of meals, and/or the actual physical activity regimen. Management issues for type 1 people with diabetes may be especially challenging due to their complete lack of ability to make metabolic adjustments to manage fuel homeostasis. PWD who are in good metabolic control and without serious complications may be able to freely participate in recreational and competitive exercise, but those with certain diabetes co-morbidities will require further assessment.

General Guidelines for Physical Activity

In general, appropriate entry-level activities for most people that are unlikely to have adverse consequences beyond sore muscles are walking, yard work, and dancing. Additional time should be added to an exercise program as the fitness level improves, but patients should be advised to stop exercising if pain or discomfort is experienced and to seek medical attention if the pain fails to subside. Because elevated blood sugar levels can cause excess water to be lost via the urine, PWD are at increased risk for developing dehydration. In addition, thirst centers in the brain are not activated until a 1 percent body water loss has occurred. It is, therefore, necessary to assure that exercise be initiated in a hydrated state and that a fluid consumption schedule be established during exercise (S. Colberg, R. Sigal and B. Fernhall et al. 2010). Table 2.2 contains basic fluid guidelines for physical activity.

Fueling the body prior to the activity and replenishing it after the activity are also crucial. Eating a meal or snack within two hours prior to exercise increases energy levels and results in an increased number of calories burned. Glycogen stores need to be replenished post-exercise, and the muscular microtears that occur with sustained activity need to be repaired within 30 minutes after exercise. During exercise lasting longer than 45 to 60 minutes, supplemental fluids and calories may be

Table 2.2 Fluid consumption schedule for physical activity (Kundrat and Rockwell 2008)

Fluid Consumption Schedule For Physical Activity		
Timing of Activity	Amount of Fluid to Consume	Note
Before Activity	16–20 ounces	Consume 2 hours prior
During Activity	8 ounces every 15 minutes	For activity lasting >1 hour, replace sodium and carbohydrate
After Activity	24 ounces for every pound of body weight lost during the activity	Weigh before and after activity to ensure proper rehydration

needed, as will more frequent blood sugar testing. When blood glucose remains within 70 to 150 mg/dL during exercise, muscle efficiency and performance are optimized (Dunford 2006),

(Hinnen et al 2001), (Kundrat and Rockwell 2008), (Walsh and Roberts 2000). MNT should be individualized based on the type, amount, and intensity of the exercise performed.

Physical Activity with Type 1 Diabetes

Exercise is not reported to improve glycemic control in persons with type 1 diabetes; however, the same benefits from exercise that the non-diabetic population experiences, such as decreased risk of CVD and improved sense of well-being, still apply. Thus regular physical activity should be encouraged in individuals with type 1 diabetes (Franz et al. 2010). It is important to note that research regarding the benefits and risks of physical activity on this population is limited. Participation in exercise may pose challenges for a person with type 1 diabetes. If a person with type 1 diabetes has a minimal amount of insulin available due to inadequate insulin therapy, the secretion of catecholamines and glucagon can cause high blood glucose levels during exercise, and if untreated, can lead to the accumulation of ketone bodies and cause diabetic ketoacidosis. It is not necessary to postpone exercise based simply on hyperglycemia as long as the patient feels well and as long as urine and blood ketones are negative. On the opposite end of the spectrum, if the person with type 1 diabetes has excessive insulin onboard, severe hypoglycemia can occur during the activity (ADA, 2013), (S. Colberg, R. Sigal and B. Fernhall et al. 2010). For this reason, it is imperative that all people with type 1 diabetes check their blood sugar before activities and always carry some form of rapid acting glucose (e.g., glucose tablets, juice) to treat hypoglycemia.

It has been reported that participation in continuous moderate-intensity exercise (aerobic activity between 40 and 59 percent of maximum oxygen uptake or 55 to 69 percent maximal heart rate) causes an increase in the risk of hypoglycemia, both during and up to 31 hours following the cessation of an activity. Additionally, during sustained high-intensity exercise (approximately 15 minutes at >80 percent of maximum oxygen uptake), a progressive rise in blood glucose levels can occur (Franz et al. 2010). In this case, with high hyperglycemia caused by vigorous activity, additional insulin should only be added after the individual's response to vigorous activity is studied on several occasions (Franz et al. 2010). A reduction in insulin dosage is the preferred method to prevent hypoglycemia when exercise is planned. For unplanned exercise, additional carbohydrate is generally required, such that a 70-kg person would need an additional 10 to 15 grams carbohydrate per hour of moderate intensity physical activity, and more if intense activity occurs (ADA, 2008).

Physical Activity with Type 2 Diabetes

Structured exercise interventions of at least eight weeks duration have been shown to lower HbA1c by an average of 0.66 percent in people with type 2 diabetes, even with no significant change in body mass index (ADA, 2013). Higher levels of exercise intensity are associated with greater improvements in HbA1c and in fitness (ADA, 2015). For adults over the age of 18, the accumulation of 150 minutes of moderate-intensity aerobic physical activity (40 to 60 percent of maximal oxygen uptake or 50 to 70 percent of maximum heart rate) per week with no more than two consecutive days between bouts of aerobic activity, in addition to resistance/strength training that involve all major muscle groups three times per week on nonconsecutive days is recommended (ADA, 2013), (S. Colberg, R. Sigal and B. Fernhall et al. 2010), (Franz et al. 2010), (Sigal et al. 2004). In a meta-analysis of eight randomized controlled trials and 18 observational studies, people who used pedometers increased their physical activity by 27 percent over baseline. In this analysis, having a goal (e.g., taking 10,000 steps per day) was as an important predictor of increased physical activity (S. Colberg, R. Sigal and B. Fernhall et al. 2010).

Independent of weight loss, both aerobic exercise and resistance training have been found to improve glycemic control and reduce cardiovascular disease risk factors. For those individuals already exercising at moderate intensity, to obtain even greater benefits in glycemic control and aerobic fitness, increasing the intensity even more is recommended. For adults over the age of 65 and for those with disabilities, the adult guidelines should be followed if possible, or if not possible, individuals should be encouraged to be as physically active as they are able (ADA, 2013). In older men with type 2 diabetes, progressive resistance exercise improves insulin sensitivity to the same or even greater extent as aerobic exercise. Clinical trials have provided strong evidence for the HbA1c-lowering value of resistance training and for an additive benefit of combined aerobic and resistance exercise (ADA, 2013).

Overall, the improvement in insulin sensitivity and the decrease risk for cardiovascular disease (e.g., through reduced LDL levels) and all-cause mortality has been shown with appropriate physical activity (Franz et al. 2010). No more than two consecutive days should pass without physical activity, in order to achieve long-term glycemic control (Franz et al. 2010), (Sigal et al. 2004). Before undertaking exercise that is more intense than brisk walking, sedentary persons with type 2 diabetes should consult a primary care practitioner (PCP). Electrocardiogram (ECG) exercise stress testing for asymptomatic individuals at low risk of CVD is not recommended but may be indicated for those who are at high risk (S. Colberg, R. Sigal and B. Fernhall et al. 2010). The general recommendations for diabetes from the American Diabetes Association Standards of Care in Diabetes 2015 are listed in Table 2.3.

Table 2.3 Physical activity and diabetes guideline recommendations (ADA, 2015)

Physical Activity and Diabetes Guideline Recommendations
Children with diabetes or prediabetes should be encouraged to engage in at least 60 minutes of physical activity each day.
Adults with diabetes should be advised to perform at least 150 minutes per week of moderate-intensity aerobic physical activity (50–70% of maximum heart rate), spread over at least 3 days/week with no more than 2 consecutive days without exercise.
Evidence supports that all individuals, including those with diabetes, should be encouraged to reduce sedentary time, particularly by breaking up extended amounts of time (>90 minutes) spent sitting.
In the absence of contraindications, adults with type 2 diabetes should be encouraged to perform resistance training at least twice per week.

References

Academy of Nutrition and Dietetics. 2011. "ADA diabetes type 1 and 2 evidence-based nutrition practice guidelines for adults." *Evidence Analysis Library.* http://andevidencelibrary.com. Accessed May 5 2012.

American Diabetes Association. 2015. "Standards of Medical Care in Diabetes - 2015." *Diabetes Care* 38(1).

___. 2015a. "Classification and diagnosis of diabetes. Sec. 2. in Standards of Medical Care in Diabetes - 2015." *Diabetes Care*, S8–S16.

___. 2015b. *Hypoglycemia (Low Blood Sugar).* http://www.diabetes.org /living-with-diabetes/treatment-and-care/blood-glucose-control/ hypoglycemia-low-blood.html. Accessed September 15, 2015.

___. 2014. *Statistics About Diabetes.* http://www.diabetes.org/diabetes-basics/statistics/. Accessed September 14, 2015.

___. 2014a. *All About Prediabetes - English.* http://professional.diabetes .org/PatientEducationLibraryDetail.aspx?pmlPath=All_About_Predi abetes_24dee6ff-cbf0-4a55-80b7-9d5d29de0bd7&pmlName=All_ About_Prediabetes.pdf&pmlId=101&pmlTitle=All%20About%20P rediabetes%20-%20English&utm_source=dorg&utm_medium=On line&utm_content=prediabetesd&utm_campaign=pem&s_src=vanit y&s_subsrc=dorg. Accessed September 14, 2015.

___. 2013. "Standards of Medical Care in Diabetes - 2013." *Diabetes Care* 36(Suppl 1): S11–66.

___. 2008. "Nutrition recommendations and interventions for diabetes: A position statement of the American Diabetes Association." *Diabetes Care* 31(Suppl 1): S61–S78.

___.2002. "Be prepared: Sick day management." *Diabetes Spectrum* 15(54).

Cefalu, WT, JE Gerich, and D LeRoith. 2004. *Council for Advancement of Diabetes Research & Education (CADRE) Handbook of Diabetes Management.* New York, NY: Medical Information Press2.

Centers for Disease Control and Prevention. 2014. *New CDC Diabetes Report.* http://www.cdc.gov/media/DPK/2014/dpk-diabetes-report.html. Accessed September 14, 2015.

Chavez, JA and SA Summers. 2003. "Characterizing the effects of saturated fatty acids on insulin signaling and ceramide and diacylglycerol accumulation in 3T3-L1 adipocytes and C2C12 myotubes." *Archives of Biochemistry and Biophysics* 419 (2): 102–109.

Colberg, S, RJ Sigal, B Fernhall, JG Regensteiner, B Blissmer, R Rubin, and B Braun. 2010. "Exercise and type 2 diabetes: The American College of Sports Medicine and the American Diabetes Association: Joint position statement." *Diabetes Care 33* (12): e147–e167.

Dunford, M. 2006. *Sports Nutrition: A Practice Manual for Professionals.* 4th ed. Chicago, IL: American Dietetic Association.

Estruck, R, RE Salas-Salvado, and et al PREDIMED Study Investigators. 2013. "Primary prevention of cardiovascular disease with a Mediterranean diet." *New England Journal of Medicine* 368: 1279–1290.

Franz, MD, JP Bantle, CA Beebe, JD Brunzell, JL Chiasson, and A Garg. 2003. "Evidence-based nutrition principles and recommendations for the treatment nad prevention of diabetes and related complications." *Diabetes Care* 26 (Suppl 1): S51–S61.

Franz, MJ, MA Powers, C Leontos, LA Holzmeister, K Kulkarni, A Monk, and E Gradwell. 2010. "The evidence for medical nutrition therapy for type 1 and type 2 diabetes in adults." *Journal of the American Dietetic Association* 110: 1852–1889.

Hinnen, DA, DW Guthrie, BP Childs, and RA Guthrie. 2001. "Pattern management of blood glucose." In *A Core Curriculum for Diabetes Education,* by MJ Franz, 173–197. Chicago, IL: American Association of Diabetes Educators.

International Diabetes Federation. 2014. *Risk Factors.* http://www.idf.org/about-diabetes/risk-factors. Accessed September 14, 2015.

Kodama, S, K Saito, S Tanaka, M Maki, Y Yachi, M Sato, and H Sone. 2009. "Influence of fat and carbohydrate proportions on the metabolic profile of people with type 2 diabetes: a meta-analysis." *Diabetes Care* 32 (5): doi: 10.2337/dc08-1716.

Kundrat, S, and M Rockwell. 2008. *Sports Dietetics: Practiced, Proven, and Tested Manual.* Nutrition on the Move, Inc.

National Institutes of Health, Medline Plus. 2014a. *Fiber.* http://www.nlm.nih.gov/medlineplus/ency/article/002470.htm. Accessed September 15, 2015.

National Institutes of Health, Medline Plus. 2014b. *Gestational Diabetes.* https://www.nlm.nih.gov/medlineplus/ency/article/000896.htm. Accessed September 15, 2015.

Post, RE, AG Mainous, DE King, and KN Simpson. 2012. "Dietary fiber for the treatment of type 2 diabetes mellitus: a meta-analysis." *Journnal of the American Board of Family Medicine* 25(1): 16–23.

Sigal, RJ, GP Kenny, DH Wasserman, and C Castaneda-Sceppa. 2004. "Physical activity/exercise and type 2 diabetes." *Diabetes Care* 27: 2518–39.

Walsh, J, and R Roberts. 2000. "Exercise." In *Pumping Insulin,* by J Walsh and R Roberts, 157–168. San Diego, CA: Torrey Pines.

Westman, EC, RD Feinman, JC Mavropoulos, MC Vernon, JS Volek, WS Yancy, and SD Phinney. 2007. "Low-carbohydrate nutrition and metabolism." *American Journal of Clinical Nutrition* 86(2): 276–284.

Wheeler, ML, and FX Pi-Sunyer. 2008. "Carbohydrate issues: type and amount." *Journal of the American Dietetic Association* 108: S34–S39.

CHAPTER 3

Metabolic Stress and Critical Illness, Cancer, and HIV/AIDS

Chapter Abstract

When the body undergoes stress and endures disease or injury, changes to the chemical environment impact nutritional status. Metabolic stress alters the metabolic rate, heart rate, blood pressure, hormonal status, and the body's ability to metabolize nutrients. Nutrient needs at this stage are often so high that the metabolically stressed, critically ill patient is unable to meet needs through oral intake alone and nutrition support becomes an integral part of the treatment plan.

In respiratory distress, problems arise that disrupt the process of exchange of gases between the air and blood. Respiratory distress results in a lowered oxygen supply in the blood and a rise in carbon dioxide levels. Increased carbon dioxide in the blood can disrupt breathing such that it impacts and interferes with food intake. Weight and optimal nutrition status are often casualties of both metabolic and respiratory distress.

The arenas of cancer and HIV/AIDS present separate but unique nutritional challenges that may range from optimizing the diet to lower cancer risk to manipulating diet to manage treatment side effects or treating chronic diseases. This chapter addresses the evidence-based nutrition therapies indicated in the prevention, treatment, and management of metabolic and pulmonary stress, and critical illness, cancer, and HIV/AIDS.

Metabolic Stress and Critical Illness

Starvation and metabolic stress result in deviations from normal nutrient metabolism that alters individual nutrient needs. A chronically starved patient with mild metabolic stress experiences a reduction in resting metabolic rate of somewhere between 10 to 30 percent (Heimburger 2015). This reduction in resting metabolic rate is the body's response to lowered energy intake that leads to a decrease in overall energy needs. In starvation, with the absence of adequate glucose from carbohydrate, the body makes alterations to utilize fat as a primary source of fuel. Lipolysis—the process of breaking down of fat for fuel—occurs as the body is adapting to conserve lean muscle mass and to prevent valuable protein loss in the absence of adequate intake. Unless this process is interrupted with the gradual resumption of normal nutrition, the chronically starved individual will eventually develop anorexia and/or cachexia.

Risk for malnutrition increases when patients experience two or more of the following conditions: inadequate calorie intake, weight loss, changes to body composition such as fat and muscle loss, accumulation of fluid or reduced grip strength (AND, 2015a). In the metabolically stressed population, malnutrition occurs when infection, traumatic injury, sepsis, or chronic inflammatory illness increase nutrient needs beyond the individual's ability to meet those needs. In metabolic stress, nutrient needs are so high that they are often unable to be met with oral intake alone, and in these cases, nutrition support becomes an integral component of treatment.

Determining Energy Needs

Energy needs are significantly elevated in metabolic stress. As compared to the healthy state, resting energy expenditure (REE) in sepsis may increase by 50 to 80 (and include urinary nitrogen excretion loads of up to 30 grams per day due to muscle catabolism and impaired protein synthesis) (Barbour, Barbour and Hermann 2015). Indirect calorimetry is the preferred method for determining energy needs for a critically ill patient. Indirect calorimetry has been shown to be more accurate than energy estimations made from predictive equations. Critically ill patients should be allowed to rest for 30 minutes prior to the measurement of resting metabolic rate. Although indirect calorimetry is the gold standard in determining energy needs, when unavailable, predictive equations may suffice for the critically ill. Predictive equations tend to be less reliable for obese patients. In the case of critical illness and obesity (BMI >30), The American Society for Parenteral and Enteral Nutrition (A.S.P.E.N.) recommends permissive underfeeding (hypocaloric feeding) with enteral nutrition. Permissive underfeeding may be associated with lower mortality rates than targeted feedings (Arabi et al. 2011). In permissive underfeeding, calories should not exceed 60 to 70 percent of target energy requirements, or 11 to 14 kcal/kg actual body weight per day (22 to 25 kcal/kg ideal body weight per day) (McClave et al. 2009). Table 3.1 contains predictive equations for the critically ill patient.

Table 3.1 Predictive equations for the critically ill. Abbreviations: PSU, Penn State University; RMR, resting metabolic rate; VE, minute ventilation in L/min; Tmax, maximum daily temperature in Celsius (AND, 2015a)

Condition	Equation
Non-obese, mechanically ventilated	PSU 2003b RMR = Mifflin (0.96) + VE (31) + Tmax (167) − 6,212
Obese, mechanically ventilated, younger than 60 years	PSU 2003b RMR = Mifflin (0.96) + VE (31) + Tmax (167) − 6,212
Obese, mechanically ventilated older than 60 years	PSU 2010 RMR = Mifflin (0.71) + VE (64) + Tmax (85) − 3,085
Mifflin equation – used in PSU (above)	RMR males = 10 × weight (kg) + 6.25 × height (cm) − 5 × age (y) + 5 RMR females = 10 × weight (kg) + 6.25 × height (cm) − 5 × age (y) − 161
Obese	11–14 kcal/kg actual weight 22–25 kcal/kg ideal body weight

Determining Protein Needs

Protein needs are certainly heightened during critical illness, although no consensus or evidence exists to suggest the best method for determining protein needs. Protein needs are generally assumed to be in the 1.2 to 2.0 g/kg/day range for metabolically stressed patients (AND, 2015a). A.S.P.E.N. guidelines recommend protein needs in the 1.2 to 2.0 g/kg/day range for those with BMI < 30, and acknowledge that protein needs may be even higher in cases of burns or multi-traumas (McClave et al. 2009). The Dietary Reference Intake (DRI) for healthy adults for protein is 0.8 g/kg/day (Institute of Medicine 2005). General guidelines suggest increasing protein include:

- 20 to 25 percent of total calories for stressed patients and those with burns
- 1.2 to 2.0 g/kg actual weight if BMI < 30 (but may be higher in burn patients)
- 2.5 g/kg/day in early post-operative burn patients, up to 4 g/kg/day during flow period
- 2.50 to 2.5 g/kg/day for continuous renal replacement therapy
- ≥2.0 g/kg ideal body weight if BMI 30 to 40 and hypocaloric feeding used
- ≥2.5 g/kg ideal body weight if BMI >40 and hypocaloric feeding used (AND, 2015a)

Determining Fluid Needs

Fluid needs in critical care are individualized based on factors that include volume depletion, degree of endothelial injury and capillary leak, and varying levels of cardiac and renal function (AND, 2015a). General fluid guidelines are estimated at 30 ml/kg/day, but hypovolemia, renal status, and cardiac function all mandate individualization of therapy. It is unlikely that enteral formulas alone will meet fluid needs, and additional water via oral, intravenous, or enteral routes is most often required to meet needs.

Nutrition Support in Critical Illness

The timely initiation of aggressive nutrition support helps maximize outcomes in critically ill patients. "Timely" is key and a primary nutrition intervention should be initiation of enteral nutrition early on at the 24 to 48 hour mark to attenuate the stress response. Feeds are started at 10 to 30 ml/hr and gradually advanced to goal rates within the next 48 to 72 hours (AND, 2015a). A.S.P.E.N. guidelines recommend achieving 50 to 65 percent of goal nutrition intake by the end of the first week. After the end of the seven to ten days, if enteral feeds are insufficient to meet total calorie needs, consider initiating supplemental parenteral nutrition (PN).

In patients with a functioning gut, early initiation of enteral nutrition (EN) helps to maintain gut integrity, reduces oxidative stress, and regulates systemic immunity (Heyland and McClave, Chapter 11. Nutrition in the Critically Ill. 2005). Gastric access for EN is preferred, but if stomach feedings are not tolerated, duodenal or jejunal access is appropriate when gastric residuals are ≥200 ml on two or more occasions despite the use of prokinetic agents (McClave et al. 2009). The head of the bed should be elevated 45 degrees to prevent aspiration in patients receiving tube feedings. Formulas are preferably high in protein, low in total fat, with at least 25 percent of fat coming from medium-chain triglyceride (MCT), and the formula should contain at least 100 percent of the daily recommended intake DRI of vitamins and minerals as well as adequate amounts of soluble dietary fiber. The Academy of Nutrition and Dietetics makes limited recommendations regarding immunonutrition formulas. The Canadian guideline, guidelines from A.S.P.E.N. and European Society for Parenteral and Enteral nutrition all give more favorable recommendations for these types of formulas based on more recent research findings (AND, 2015a), (Heyland, Dhaliwal et al. 2003), (McClave et al. 2009), (Kreymann et al. 2006).

For optimal outcomes, nutrition support and the tolerance of EN or PN should be closely monitored. Complications of nutrition support may be gastrointestinal in nature, may increase the risk of aspiration, and can result in fluid imbalances or hyperglycemia. Diarrhea is the most common complication of EN and occurs as a result of medication, use of hypertonic solutions, or antibiotic use that kills beneficial bacteria. The primary approach to managing diarrhea with EN should be a review of the medication list. Initiation of supplemental soluble fiber may also be beneficial.

Nutrition in Pulmonary Stress

Nutrition in Acute Respiratory Distress Syndrome

Pulmonary stress initiates a hypermetabolic, catabolic state. Even when overweight with acute respiratory distress syndrome (ARDS), weight loss should be prevented (AND, 2015a). A secondary goal of nutrition therapy is to prevent overfeeding, which leads to excessive CO_2 production that further depresses respiratory function. Protein needs in ARDS and acute lung injury (ALI) are estimated to range from 1.5 to 2.0 g/kg body weight per day (Schwartz 1998). Fluid needs are normal for ARDS and ALI, unless another underlying condition dictates a fluid restriction.

There is no general consensus regarding the use of immune-enhancing formulas in the enterally fed patient with ARDS and ALI. A number of studies suggest that these patients should receive enteral formulas enriched with dietary fish oil containing eicosapentaenoic acid, borage oil containing gamma-linolenic acid, and higher levels of antioxidant vitamins (Singer et al. 2006), (Pontes-Arruda, Aragao and Albuquerque 2006), (Gadek et al. 1999). The Academy of Nutrition and Dietetics' evidence analysis project on the topic states the opposite, maintaining that,

> "Immune-enhancing enteral nutrition is not recommended for *routine* use in critically ill patients in the intensive care unit. Immune-enhancing enteral nutrition is not associated with reduced infectious complications, length of stay, reduced cost of medical care, days on mechanical ventilation, or mortality in moderately to less severely ill intensive care unit patients. Their use may be associated with increased mortality in severely ill intensive care unit patients, although adequately-powered trials evaluating this have not been conducted. For the trauma patient,

it is not recommended to routinely use immune-enhancing enteral nutrition, as its use is not associated with reduced mortality, reduced length of stay, reduced infectious complications or fewer days on mechanical ventilation" (AND, 2012).

Nutrition in Chronic Obstructive Pulmonary Disease

Both underweight and unintentional weight loss are common problems for people with chronic obstructive pulmonary disease (COPD). Patients with COPD who are underweight may experience associated nutrition-related problems as their condition greatly increases energy requirements. The work required for breathing in COPD may be 10 to 20 times that of a person with normal lung function. Energy expenditure is elevated as the body works harder to breathe, combats chronic infection, and experiences altered metabolism. Energy expenditure is also affected by participation in pulmonary rehabilitation exercise programs, which can lead to increased fatigue at meal time, further decrease intake, and increase weight loss. Risk for COPD-related death doubles with weight loss, and BMI of <20 kg/m^2 may be seen in up to 30 percent of individuals with COPD. Energy needs are even higher during COPD exacerbation. The most accurate way to determine caloric needs in these patients is through the use of indirect calorimetry.

Feeding goals for COPD focus on achieving maximum nutrition with minimal effort and fatigue. Nutrition practitioners should encourage patients to eat slowly, biting and chewing methodically, and breathing deeply while they eat. Placing utensils down between bites can help appropriately pace food intake. Encourage patients to select foods that are easy to chew and prepare, and opt for five or six small meals per day. Encourage them to drink liquids between meals or at the end of meals to conserve valuable space in the stomach for food. Also encourage them to sit upright while eating and avoid lying down immediately after meals in order to reduce pressure on the lungs.

While the calorie needs are significantly higher in the COPD population, the distribution of macronutrients does not differ much from that of healthy people. Specific vitamin and mineral considerations involve vitamin C and sodium. As with smokers, COPD patients who

Table 3.2 Nutrition intervention strategies for COPD (AND, 2015a)

Nutrition Intervention Strategies for COPD
Liberalize diet to encourage oral intake within the parameters of medical priorities.
Provide small, frequent, mini-meals and snacks to help compensate for shortness of breath and reduced oxygen supply to GI tract.
Choose foods that are easy to chew, swallow, and digest.
Utilize easy to prepare whole grains, fruits, and vegetables to achieve fiber intake goals.
Include nutrient-dense nutrition supplements or shakes between meals to meet calorie goals.
Supplement diet with vitamin-mineral supplements.
Exercise appropriate sitting posture and practice sequencing of breathing to increase ease of swallowing and eating.
Discourage elimination of milk from the diet; milk is unrelated to mucus production despite common beliefs otherwise.

smoke have increased vitamin C needs of 35 mg per day above the healthy, non-smoking population, meaning that male adult smokers need 125 mg vitamin C per day and female adult smokers need 105 mg vitamin C total per day (IM, 2000). For patients with cor pulmonale and fluid retention, consider limiting both sodium and fluid. If on diuretic therapy, the COPD patient should increase dietary potassium intake. Individuals with COPD are advised to undergo bone mineral density screening, as they are at increased risk for developing osteoporosis (AND, 2015a). By far, the greatest challenge in nutrition care for COPD, especially in underweight people, is consuming adequate calories. Table 3.2 contains a list of helpful nutrition intervention strategies for people with COPD to maximize their calorie intake.

Cancer

Nutrition and diet play roles in both the prevention and management of cancer. Although the medical community does not entirely understand the intricacies of how each aspect of the diet affects the initiation and progress of every type of cancer, there is a general agreement that a diet rich in plant foods, and one that is low in animal foods, seems to protect against certain types of cancer. This is also the preferred diet for most people undergoing cancer treatment. While well-balanced diets can help lower risk, there is no one known dietary approach that will outright prevent cancer. Research indicates that the combination of a healthy diet along with a physically active lifestyle and maintenance of a healthy weight are the cornerstones of cancer prevention (WCFR and AICR, 2007).

Nutrition and Cancer Prevention

The World Cancer Research Fund (WCFR) and the American Institute for Cancer Research (AICR) suggest that one in three cancer cases can be prevented through changes in diet and lifestyle. The WCRF/AICR maintains that the tenets of cancer prevention are an optimal diet, adequate levels of physical activity, and a healthy weight.

Long before the USDA adopted MyPlate and plate-based methods of meal planning, AICR endorsed their own plate method called "The New American Plate." The New American Plate model suggests that two-thirds of the plate should be fruits, vegetables, and whole grains, while less than one-third should be lean animal protein. For individuals who do consume animal foods, lean or low fat sources of animal protein are preferred. In their report, *Food, Nutrition, Physical Activity, and the Prevention of Cancer: a Global Perspective*, the AICR recommends the following for preventing cancer:

- Eating mostly plant-based foods, which are low in energy density
- Being physically active
- Maintaining a healthy weight (by following the two steps above, as well as reducing portion size)

In addition to eating more plants and less animals, it appears that limiting salt, alcohol intake, and foods and drinks that promote weight gain, and achieving a healthy weight along with physical activity may protect against the development of certain types of cancer (WCRF and AICR, 2007). More specific dietary recommendations for cancer prevention include:

- Eating five servings of non-starchy fruits and vegetables per day
- Eating relatively unprocessed grains and/or legumes for every meal
- Limiting refined starchy foods
- Minimizing processed meat, and if one does eat red meat, limiting it to no more than 18 oz. of red meat per week
- Limiting consumption of alcohol to one drink per day for women and two drinks per day for men
- Limiting salt intake to less than 6 grams (2,400 mg sodium) per day
- Avoiding sugary drinks and consume fast foods sparingly, if at all

In addition to being overweight and consuming a high-animal foods diet, there are other factors that can increase the risk of developing cancer. Additional risk factors include excessive sunlight exposure, cigarette smoking or tobacco use, under-vaccination, and exposure to environmental pollutants. Table 3.3 outlines the cancer prevention guidelines from the World Cancer Research Fund and American Institute for Cancer Research

Table 3.3 Cancer prevention guidelines from the World Cancer Research Fund and American Institute for Cancer Research (WCRF and AICR, 2007)

Cancer Prevention Guidelines	
Body Fatness	Be as lean as possible within the normal range of body weight.
Physical Activity	Be physically active as a part of everyday life.
Foods and Drinks That Promote Weight Gain	Limit consumption of energy-dense foods and avoid sugary drinks.
Plant Foods	Eat mostly foods of plant origin.
Animal Foods	Limit intake of red meat and avoid processed meat.
Alcoholic Drinks	Limit alcoholic drinks.
Preservation, Processing, and Preparation	Limit salt intake and avoid moldy cereals (grains) or pulses (legumes).

Cancer Prevention Guidelines	
Dietary Supplements	Aim to meet nutritional needs through diet alone.
Breastfeeding	Mother should breastfeed when possible and children should be breastfed when possible.
Cancer Survivors	Follow the recommendations for cancer prevention.

Antioxidants and Cancer

Antioxidants are compounds that have the potential to block the activity of other chemicals called free radicals. Free radicals are highly reactive chemicals that have the potential to harm cells. The damage done to the cells, particularly to the DNA of the cells, may play a role in the development of cancer and other diseases (NCI, 2014). Antioxidants are sometimes called free radical scavengers. While some antioxidants can be made by the body, others are obtained from the diet. Examples of dietary sources of antioxidants include:

- Beta-carotene
- Lycopene
- Vitamin A
- Vitamin C
- Vitamin E

The mineral selenium is sometimes considered a dietary antioxidant, although the antioxidant activity of proteins that contain selenium is more likely to provide the antioxidant activity than the element on its own (Davis, Tsuji and Milner 2012).

Because of the role that free radicals play in the development of cancer and due to the potential for antioxidants to block this activity, people are curious about using antioxidant supplements for cancer prevention and treatment. In a review of nine clinical trials conducted to study the effect of antioxidant supplementation on cancer prevention, the National Cancer Institute (NCI) has determined that, "Overall, these nine randomized controlled clinical trials did not provide evidence that dietary antioxidant supplements are beneficial in primary cancer prevention"

(NCI 2014). The U.S. Preventive Services Task Force (USPSTF) has also concluded that there is no clear benefit for the use of antioxidant supplements in the prevention of cancer (Fortmann et al. 2013). Antioxidant supplements also do not appear to be useful for people who already have cancer, and in some cases, outcomes were actually worse, especially for those who were smokers (Lawenda et al. 2008).

Nutrition and Cancer Treatment

For people already diagnosed with cancer, healthy eating and maintaining optimal nutrition can help maintain strength, keep body tissue healthy, and fight against infection. Because cancer can change the way your body utilizes certain nutrients, additional vitamin and/or mineral supplements or alterations to the diet may be recommended as a part of a cancer patient's treatment plan. Cancer, its side effects, and the effects of treatment such as chemotherapy and radiation can also change the body's relationship with food and the ability to ingest food (NCI 2014a). Some common nutrition-related side effects include:

- Anorexia (loss of appetite)
- Mouth sores or dry mouth
- Trouble swallowing
- Nausea and vomiting
- Diarrhea and constipation
- Pain, depression, and anxiety

Cancer treatments and medications can interfere with the way food tastes and smells. These, along with the side effects listed above, can all contribute to a reduced intake and resultant malnutrition. Malnutrition may worsen as the cancer advances, making it increasingly difficult for the person with cancer to adequately eat the amount and types of foods needed to help keep the body strong during treatment. Table 3.4 offers high calorie, high protein recommendations for meeting increased needs during cancer treatment.

Table 3.4 High fat, high calorie ideas to increase intake in cancer patients

High Fat, High Calorie Ideas to Increase Intake in Cancer Patients
Add oils, butter, or margarine to foods, soups, and casseroles.
Sauté vegetables and meats in oil.
Use full fat condiments such as mayonnaise or salad dressings and cream cheese.
Try half-and-half and cream, whole milk.
Snack on nuts, cheese, eggs, or add high fat meats to menu items.
Drink oral supplements between meals.
Consume beverages between meals to increase calorie intake from foods at meals.

Determining Protein Needs

Alongside a reduction in muscle protein synthesis, protein turnover rates increase in cancer. Evidence-based guidelines state that protein needs are elevated beyond the standard 0.8 g/kg RDA for those with head and neck cancer, in those undergoing radiation therapy, and in those with hematological malignancies undergoing allogeneic hematopoietic stem cell transplants. Protein needs are 0.8 to 1.0 g/kg for normal maintenance, 1.0 to 1.2 g/kg for non-stressed patient with cancer, 1.2 to 1.5 g/kg for those undergoing treatment, 1.5 to 2.0 g/kg for stem cell transplant, and 1.5 to 2.5 g/kg for those with protein-losing enteropathies or wasting (AND, 2015b), (Hurst and Gallagher 2006). Protein should be limited to 0.5 to 0.8 g/kg with hepatic or renal compromise, when BUN is approaching 100 mg/dL, or in light of elevated ammonia levels (Cohen 2011). Dietetics practitioners can also request labs for serum proteins such as albumin, prealbumin, and transferrin to monitor nutrition status. C-reactive protein (CRP) may also be a useful biomarker, as it is sensitive to inflammation and may serve as a precursor to cachexia.

Soy and Breast Cancer

Many people wonder about the effect of soy on certain types of cancer, including breast cancer. Soy contains compounds that act like estrogen in the body. The National Cancer Institute has conducted and evaluated research that has found the following (NCI, 2014a):

- Some studies show that eating soy foods may decrease the risk of having breast cancer.
- Taking soy supplements in the form of powders or pills has not been shown to prevent breast cancer.
- Avoiding soy foods in the diet after being diagnosed with breast cancer has not been shown to keep the breast cancer from coming back.

Management of Nutrition-Related Treatment Side Effects

Cancer treatment can be as devastating to the body as the disease itself. Side effects from chemotherapy or radiation treatment may alter nutrition and cause nausea and vomiting, constipation, inflammation of the mucosa and mouth (mucositis and stomatitis), smell and taste alterations (dysgeusia), dry mouth (xerostomia), early satiety, and cancer cachexia-anorexia syndrome.

Nausea and Vomiting

Six to eight small meals and snacks per day, spread out over the day can help the person undergoing cancer treatment meet his or her needs despite increasing levels of fatigue and elevated nutrient needs. Some patients find that ingesting bland, dry foods, such as saltines, before getting out of bed in the morning may minimize nausea and vomiting. Cancer patients are advised to avoid foods that have strong odors; many find that cold foods are better tolerated than hot temperature and spicy foods. Fried foods, greasy foods, and high fat foods may all trigger nausea and vomiting. Sipping on juices, sports drinks, ginger ale, or clear soda throughout the day will help avoid dehydration while also providing calories. Prolonged vomiting can induce dehydration; during bouts of vomiting, sip on clear liquids as much as possible, aiming to drink an additional half to one cup of liquid for each episode of vomiting. People with cancer who are experiencing nausea and vomiting should work to create a peaceful eating place that is devoid of distractions, and one that is well ventilated to prevent accumulation of food and cooking odors (Eldridge and Hamilton 2004).

Diarrhea and Constipation

If cancer treatment is causing constipation, the same guidelines for minimizing constipation in healthy population are recommended. Those with constipation should work to increase fluid intake, whole grains and fiber intake from fruits, vegetables, and legumes. Increasing physical activity can also help alleviate constipation, although exercise may be contraindicated or overly exhausting during treatment. When necessary, consider a bulking agent or over-the-counter fiber supplement. However, be mindful that fiber-containing foods may be filling and may reduce overall intake. As such, patients should be closely monitored to ensure they are ingesting sufficient calories and not losing weight.

For diarrhea, investigate what may be making diarrhea worse. Medication adjustments or removal or certain supplements may help alleviate diarrhea. Limiting juices, particularly those with sorbitol, can help decrease diarrhea. Foods or beverages that contain sugar alcohols (such as mannitol, sorbitol, and xylitol) will likely make diarrhea worse. On the other hand, sipping on low sugar, clear liquids can help rehydrate. During active diarrhea, encourage fluid intake of at least one cup of fluid for each loose bowel movement. Provide intravenous fluids if dehydration risk is imminent and recommend antidiarrheal medications when appropriate. Probiotic supplements may be helpful in those whose diarrhea is related to altered microflora counts from antibiotic use. General dietary precautions in diarrhea are to avoid foods with excess fat, lactose, and simple sugars in them (AND, 2015b).

Mucositis and Stomatitis

Mucositis (inflammation of the mucus membrane of the mouth or GI tract) and stomatitis (inflammation of the mouth) both inhibit the cancer patient's ability to consume optimal nutrients. Those with inflammation of the oral cavity should avoid known irritants such as tobacco, alcohol, spicy foods, and coarse or acidic foods such as tomatoes, oranges, or other

Table 3.5 Potential supplements for use in cancer-related mucositis (Coghlin Dickson et al. 2000), (Rogers 2001), (Berger et al. 1995), (Surh and Lee 1995), (Biswal, Zakari and Ahmad 2003)

Potential Supplements for use in Cancer-Related Mucositis	
Glutamine	• May reduce mucositis during cancer therapies • Dose as 10 g glutamine 3–4 times per day • For sore mouth: swish around mouth for 1–2 minutes, swallow • Not for use with compromised renal or liver function
Chamomile	• Believed to have anti-inflammatory, antibacterial, and antifungal properties • Safe when consumed in food; inexpensive • Not definitely shown to alleviate pain when compared to placebo
Capsaicin	• Substance derived from hot pepper plant • Known analgesic properties • Postulated that repeat administration of capsaicin desensitizes and inactivates sensory neurons, giving pain relief
Honey	• Ameliorating potential for severity of mucositis for patient undergoing radiation • 20 ml pure honey 15 minutes before, 15 minutes after and 6 hours post-radiation therapy • Topical application had slight reduction in grade 3–4 mucositis with 54 percent maintaining or gaining weight

citrus foods that aggravate the tissues. Cold temperature foods may be better than hot temperature foods. Likewise, soft, moist foods may also be more acceptable than dry, rough, or coarse foods. Sucking on ice chips or popsicles can help numb the mouth area and reduce discomfort during meal times. The use of topical and/or systemic analgesics may also be helpful in pain management. The Academy of Nutrition and Dietetics recommends supplementation with zinc at levels of 220 mg two to three times per day to help improve mucositis and taste changes that occur with radiation therapy (AND, 2015b). Table 3.5 contains a list of other potentially helpful supplements used in managing mucositis.

Alterations in Taste and Smell

Cancer treatment often interferes with the normal taste and smell of foods. Foods that used to be preferred may become intolerable during chemotherapy or radiation. Metallic tastes are particularly heightened during certain cancer treatments. If oral nutrition supplements are consumed, advise the patient not to drink them from a metal can or container; instead, transfer the liquid supplement to a plastic cup, or drink it through a straw to avoid contact with the metallic vessel. Consider plastic utensils if metallic ones are bothersome. Chilled foods tend to be better tolerated than hot foods. If foods are perceived to be too sweet, consider adding sour sauces, lemon, or salt to decrease the sweetness. Marinate meats, which are high in mineral content, in fruit juice or sweet wine to disguise any potential bitter or metallic tastes. If red meats are too bitter to be palatable, consider poultry, fish, and vegetarian sources of protein as nutrient-dense alternatives (AND, 2015b). Encourage people undergoing cancer treatment to avoid eating their favorite foods unless they are feeling well; consuming favorite foods during times of illness will cause the person to associate that formerly favorite food with being sick and will slowly (or quickly) decrease the pleasure that was previously associated with eating those favorite foods.

Dry Mouth (Xerostomia)

While dry mouth (xerostomia) may be precipitated by chemotherapy agents and radiation of the oral cavity, other factors may also contribute to dry mouth, including Sjögren's syndrome, dehydration, alcohol, tobacco, medication use, poor oral hygiene, graft-versus-host disease, and the physiology of aging (Strohl 2002). Oral care protocol should be used to prevent xerostomia: rinse mouth with water and baking soda (half to one teaspoon in eight ounces of water) every two hours while awake, avoid mouthwashes that contain alcohol, and brush teeth with very soft head baby toothbrush. Maintaining good oral hygiene and using a cool mist humidifier overnight help prevent dry mouth. Avoid tobacco, alcohol, and caffeine, because they all lead to further dryness. Encourage increased fluid intake and constant sipping of water throughout the day. Other pharmacological agents that may be given prior to radiation to prevent dry mouth include saliva substitutes or artificial saliva that moisten the oral mucosa and facilitate ease of speaking, swallowing, and chewing foods (AND, 2015b). Additionally, reduce intake of sucrose-containing foods and carbohydrates in the diet that will stick to the teeth and, in turn, increase the risk of cavities.

Nutrition in HIV/AIDS

It is estimated that there are more than 1.2 million people currently living with HIV infection in the United States; and of these, roughly one in eight (12.8 percent) are unaware of their infected status. Each year in the United States, approximately 50,000 people are infected with HIV; this is down from the late 1990s when more than 3 million new infections were reported annually (CDC, 2015), (AND, 2015c). With advances in medicine that have led to the widespread use of highly active antiretroviral therapy (HAART) drugs, people with HIV/AIDS are experiencing longer lifespans. With these extended years of life, those with HIV/AIDS are increasingly more likely to succumb to the nutritional pitfalls of chronic diseases than to experience nutrient-related side effects of their condition. As such, nutrition therapy with HIV/AIDS should concentrate on the realities of existing comorbidities that are typically seen in non-infected aging groups, such as dyslipidemia, cardiovascular disease, hypertension, stroke, renal and liver disease, and diabetes.

Lipodystrophy syndrome is common in HIV infection and is characterized by high plasma triglycerides, total cholesterol, and apolipoprotein B seen in conjunction with hyperinsulinemia and hyperglycemia. In lipodystrophy syndrome, subcutaneous fat is lost in the limbs and facial region, but is redeposited in the abdomen, dorsocervical, and breast areas. Lipodystrophy affects between 33 to 75 percent of those with HIV infection who are receiving combination antiretroviral therapy (cART), and approximately 20 percent of people with HIV-associated lipodystrophy also meet the diagnostic criteria for the metabolic syndrome. Metabolic syndrome is covered in Chapter 1.

Blood lipids may be higher in HIV/AIDS because of infection, medication interaction, family history, or genetic predisposition. Individuals with elevated cholesterol and triglyceride levels are advised to follow the same general dietary guidelines recommended for heart health covered in Chapter 1.

Calorie needs are determined using many of the same factors that are relevant to the non-infected population: age, gender, disease state, nutrient status, presence or absence of opportunistic infections, inflammation, medication, or comorbidities. Resting energy expenditure may be

5 to 17 percent higher in some cases of HIV, but the energy expenditure rates of HIV patients are often similar to that of healthy individuals (AND, 2015c).

References

Academy of Nutrition and Dietetics. 2015. "Critical Illness." *Nutrition Care Manual.*. http://www.nutritioncaremanual.org. Accessed September 18, 2015.

___. 2015a. "HIV/AIDS." *Nutrition Care Manual.* http://www.nutritioncaremanual.org. Accessed September 18, 2015.

___. 2015b. "Oncology." *Nutrition Care Manual.* http://www.nutritioncaremanual.org. Accessed September 18, 2015.

___. 2015c. "Pulmonary." *Nutrition Care Manual.* http://www.nutritioncaremanual.org. Accessed September 18, 2015.

___. 2012. "Recommendations Summary: Critical Illness (CI)." *Evidence Analysis Library.* http://andevidencelibrary.com. Accessed September 18, 2015.

Arabi, YM, HM Tamim, GS Dhar, A Al-Dawood, M Al-Sultan, MH Saakijha, SH Kahoul, and R Brits. 2011. "Permissive underfeeding and intensive insulin therapy in critically ill patients: a randomized controlled trial." *The American Journal of Clinical Nutrition* 93 (3): 569–577.

Barbour, JR, EF Barbour, and VM Hermann. 2015. "Chapter 10. Surgical Metabolism & Nutrition." In *CURRENT Diagnosis & Treatment: Surgery*, by GM (Ed) Doherty.

Berger, A, M Henderson, W Nadoolman, V Duffy, D Cooper, L Saberski, and L Bartoshuk. 1995. "Oral capsaicin provides temporary relief for oral mucositis pain secondary to chemotherapy/radiation therapy." *Journal of Pain Symptom Manage* 10 (3): 243–248.

Biswal, B, A Zakari, and N Ahmad. 2003. "Topical application of honey in the management of radiation mucositis: a preliminary study." *Support Care Cancer* 11 (4): 242–248.

Centers for Disease Control and Prevention. 2015. *HIV in the United States: At a Glance.* July 1. http://www.cdc.gov/hiv/statistics/basics/ataglance.html. Accessed September 18, 2015.

Coghlin Dickson, TM, RM Wong, RS Offrin, JA Shizuru, LJ Johnston, WW Hu, KG Blume, and KE Stockerl-Goldstein. 2000. "Effect of oral glutamine supplementation during bone marrow transplantation." *Journal of Parenteral & Enteral Nutrition* 24 (2): 61–66.

Cohen, DA. 2011. "Neoplastic Disease." In *Nutrition Therapy and Pathophysiology*, by M Nelms, KP Sucher, K Lacey and SL Roth. Belmong, CA: Wadsworth.

Davis, CD, PA Tsuji, and JA Milner. 2012. "Selenoproteins and Cancer Prevention." *Annual Review of Nutrition* 32: 73–95.

Eldridge, B, and KK Hamilton. 2004. *Management of Nutrition Impact Symptoms and Educational Handouts*. Chicago: The American Dietetic Association.

Fortmann, SP, BU Burda, CA Senger, and et al. 2013. "Vitamin and mineral supplements in the primary prevention of cardiovascular disease and cancer: an updated systematic evidence review for the U.S. Preventive Services Task Force." *Annals of Internal Medicine* 159 (12): 824–34.

Gadek, JE, SJ DeMichele, MD Karlstad, ER Pacht, M Donahoe, E Albertson, C Van Hoozen, AK Weenberg, JL Nelson, and M Noursalehi. 1999. "Effect of enteral feeding with eicosapentaenoic acid, gamma-linolenic acid, and antioxidants in patients with acute respiratory distress syndrome. Enteral Nutrition in ARDS Study Group." *Critcal Care Medicine* 27: 1409–1420.

Heimburger, DC. 2015. "Chapter 97. Malnutrition and Nutritional Assessment." In *Harrison's Principles of Internal Medicine*, by DL Longo, AS Fauci, DL Kasper, SL Hauser, JL Jameson and J (Eds) Loscalzo.

Heyland, DK, and SA McClave. 2005. "Chaper 11. Nutrition in the Critically Ill." In *Principles of Crtical Care*, by JB Hall, GA Schmidt and LD (Eds) Woods.

Heyland, DK, R Dhaliwal, JW Drover, L Gramlich, and P Dodek. 2003. "Canadian clinical practice guidelines for nutrition support in mechanically ventilated, critically ill adult patients." *Journal of Parenteral & Enteral Nutrition* 27 (5): 355–73.

Hurst, JD, and AL Gallagher. 2006. "Energy, macronutrient, micronutrient, and fluid requirements." In *The Clinical Guide to Oncology Nutrition*. Chicago, IL: American Dietetic Association.

Institute of Medicine. 2005. Dietary Reference Intakes for Energy, Carbohydrate, Fiber, Fat, Fatty Acids, Cholesterol, Protein, and Amino Acids (Macronutrients). Washington, DC: National Academies Press.

___. 2000. Dietary Reference Intakes for Vitamin C, Vitamin E, Selenium, and Carotenoids. National Academies Press.

Kreymann, KG, MM Berger, NEP Deutz, M Hiesmayr, P Jolliet, G Kazandjiev, G Nitenberg, et al. 2006. "ESPEN guidelines on enteral nutrition: Intensive care." *Clinical Nutrition* 25: 210–23.

Lawenda, BD, KM Kelly, EJ Ladas, and et al. 2008. "Should supplemental antioxidant administration be avoided during chemotherapy and radiation therapy?" *Journal of the National Cancer Institute* 100 (11): 773–783.

McClave, SF, RG Martindale, VW Vanek, M McCarthy, P Roberts, B Taylor, JB Ochoa, L Napolitano, and G Cresci. 2009. "Guidelines for the Provision and Assessment of Nutrition Support Therapy in the Adult Critically Ill Patient: Society of Critical Care Medicine (SCCM) and American Society for Parenteral and Enteral Nutrition (A.S.P.E.N.)." *Journal of Parenteral & Enteral Nutrition* 33 (3): 277–316.

National Cancer Institute. 2014. *Antioxidants and Cancer Prevention.* January 16. Accessed September 18, 2015. http://www.cancer.gov /cancertopics/causes-prevention/risk-factors/diet/antioxidants-fact-sheet.

___. 2014. *Nutrition in Cancer Care (PDQ).* December 15. http://www .cancer.gov/cancertopics/pdq/supportivecare/nutrition/Patient/page1. Accessed September 18, 2015.

Pontes-Arruda, A, AM Aragao, and JD Albuquerque. 2006. "Effects of enteral feeding with eicosapentaenoic acid, gamma-linolenic acid, and antioxidants in mechanically ventilated patients with severe sepsis and septic shock." *Critical Care Medicine* 34: 2325–2333.

Rogers, B. 2001. "Mucositis in the oncology patient." *Nursing Clinics of North America* 36 (4): 745–759.

Schwartz, D. 1998. "Pulmonary failure." In *Contemporary Nutrition Support Practice: A Clinical Guide*, by LE Matarese and MM Gottschlich, 395–408. Philadelphia, PA: WB Saunders.

Singer, P, M Theilla, H Fisher, L Fibstein, E Grozovski, and J Cohen. 2006. "Benefit of an enteral diet enriched with eicosapentaenoic acid and gamma-linolenic acid in ventilated patients with acute lung injury." *Critical Care Medicine* 34: 1033–1038.

Strohl, R. 2002. "Stomatitis/xerostomia." In *Clinical Manual for the Oncology Advanced Practice Nurse*, by D Camp-Sorell and R, eds. Hawkins. Pittsburgh, PA: Oncology Nursing Press, Inc.

Surh, Y-J, and S Lee. 1995. "Capsaicin, a double-edged sword: toxicity, metabolism, and chemopreventive potential." *Life Science* 56: 1845–1855.

World Cancer Research Fund and American Institute for Cancer Research. 2007. "Second Expert Report: Food, Physical Activity & The Prevention of Cancer."

World Cancer Research Fund and American Institute for Cancer Research. 2007. "Second Expert Report: Food, Physical Activity & The Prevention of Cancer."

Index

OTHER TITLES IN OUR NUTRITION AND DIETETIC PRACTICE COLLECTION

Katie Ferraro, *Editor*

FORTHCOMING IN THIS COLLECTION

- *Diet and Disease: Nutrition for Gastrointestinal, Musculoskeletal, Hepatobiliary, Pancreatic, and Kidney Diseases* by Katie Ferraro
- *Introduction to Dietetic Practice* by Katie Ferraro
- *Dietary Supplements* by B. Bryan Haycock and Amy A. Sunderman
- *Nutrition Support* by Brenda O'Day
- *Weight Management and Obesity* by Courtney Winston Paolicelli
- *Sports Nutrition* by Kary Woodruff

Momentum Press is one of the leading book publishers in the field of engineering, mathematics, health, and applied sciences. Momentum Press offers over 30 collections, including Aerospace, Biomedical, Civil, Environmental, Nanomaterials, Geotechnical, and many others.

Momentum Press is actively seeking collection editors as well as authors. For more information about becoming an MP author or collection editor, please visit http://www.momentumpress.net/contact

Announcing Digital Content Crafted by Librarians

Momentum Press offers digital content as authoritative treatments of advanced engineering topics by leaders in their field. Hosted on ebrary, MP provides practitioners, researchers, faculty, and students in engineering, science, and industry with innovative electronic content in sensors and controls engineering, advanced energy engineering, manufacturing, and materials science.

Momentum Press offers library-friendly terms:
- perpetual access for a one-time fee
- no subscriptions or access fees required
- unlimited concurrent usage permitted
- downloadable PDFs provided
- free MARC records included
- free trials

The **Momentum Press** digital library is very affordable, with no obligation to buy in future years.

For more information, please visit **www.momentumpress.net/library** or to set up a trial in the US, please contact **mpsales@globalepress.com**.

www.ingramcontent.com/pod-product-compliance
Lightning Source LLC
Chambersburg PA
CBHW052017230326
41598CB00078B/3549